One of Us

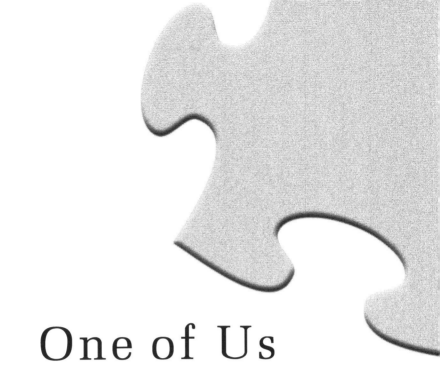

One of Us

A Family's Life with Autism

Mark Osteen

University of Missouri Press   Columbia

Copyright © 2010 by
The Curators of the University of Missouri
University of Missouri Press, Columbia, Missouri 65211
Printed and bound in the United States of America
All rights reserved
First paperback printing, 2018

Cataloging-in Publication data
available from the Library of Congress
ISBN 978-0-8262-2190-2 (paperback)

∞™ This paper meets the requirements of the
American National Standard for Permanence of Paper
for Printed Library Materials, Z39.48, 1984.

Design and composition: Jennifer Cropp
Printing and binding: Thomson-Shore, Inc.
Typefaces: Minion and Memoir

An earlier version of chapter 11 was published in *Autism and Representation,* ed. Mark Osteen (New York and London: Routledge, 2008), and is reprinted by permis-sion; chapters 12 and 15 were first published in *Weber—The Contemporary West.* Excerpts from the following are reprinted by permission: "Bye-Child," from *Opened Ground: Selected Poems 1966-1996,* by Seamus Heaney, copyright © 1998 by Seamus Heaney, reprinted by permission of Farrar, Straus, and Giroux, LLC and by Faber and Faber, Ltd.; "Death of a Young Man by Drowning," from *The Journals of Su-sanna Moodie,* by Margaret Atwood, copyright © 1976 by Oxford University Press, reprinted by permission of Houghton Mifflin Harcourt Publishing Company, all rights reserved, and with the permission of Curtis Brown Group Ltd., London, on behalf of Margaret Atwood, copyright © O. W. Toad, 1970; "Little Gidding," from *Four Quartets,* by T. S. Eliot, reprinted by permission of Faber and Faber, Ltd.; "A Martian Sends a Postcard Home," by Craig Raine, copyright © Craig Raine, 1979; "Prisoners," by Denise Levertov, from *Oblique Prayers,* copyright © 1984 by Denise Levertov, reprinted by permission of New Directions Publishing Corp.; "Spring and All, Section 1," by William Carlos Williams, from *The Collected Poems: Volume I, 1909-1939,* copyright © 1938 by New Directions Publishing Corp., reprinted by permission of New Directions Publishing Corp.

For Cameron

Contents

Acknowledgments   ix
Prologue: The Other World   1

Part One: Awakenings

1. Yankee Doodle Dandy   7
2. The News   14
3. Jabberwocky   24
4. Raw Timber   32
5. Golden Slumbers   42
6. The Thing with Feathers   51
7. Melting Down   63
8. Holding Patterns   76
9. The Red Queen's Race   86
10. Camp Wonder   99

Part Two: Refractions

11. Urinetown   125
12. The Play of Shadows   136
13. A Brief History of Stims   147
14. As Others See Us   161
15. In the Echo Chamber   172

Part Three: Emergenc(i)es

16. Fighting Words   183
17. May Day!   193
18. Departures   208
19. Returns   221
20. Nosology   234
21. Letting Go   247

Epilogue: One of Us   259
References   263
Bibliography   267

Acknowledgments

The author of a book so long in the making accrues debts to many people. Quite a few of those people—Cam's teachers, therapists, aides, and doctors—contributed immensely through their expertise and care for our son. Instead of thanking them all by name here, I've expressed our gratitude in the pages within. Below are the folks who helped directly with the manuscript.

Martha Woodmansee first suggested that I write this book; Lois Wallace provided an honest and helpful assessment of the first draft; Tracy Bernstein supplied much good advice at a later stage. I am extremely grateful to them, and to my colleagues at the Loyola University English and Writing departments, particularly June Ellis and Bryan Crockett, who read and tactfully commented on earlier versions of the manuscript. James Buckley, dean of the Loyola College of Arts and Sciences, furnished essential support both personal and financial. Big thanks are also due to Katherine Fausset for believing in this book and for suggesting the revised ending. Even bigger thanks go to my friends and fellow writers Scott Allen, Ned Balbo, and Ron Tanner for their editorial suggestions and steadfast encouragement. In addition to improving the writing in a multitude of ways, they also gave me the faith to forge on.

My greatest thanks, of course, go to Leslie. In this case, the cliché is literally true: *One of Us* wouldn't exist without her. Her courage, humor, intelligence, and love make her the heroine of this book and of my life.

What man is there of you, whom if his son ask for bread, will he give him a stone?

—Matthew 7:9

Prologue

The Other World

Today is July 4, 2000. My son Cameron turns eleven. For him, as for most kids, it's a big day. But we haven't planned a picnic, and Cam won't be playing Nintendo, soccer, or Little League baseball.

Instead, he'll spend the day watching the same videos and listening to the same songs he has enjoyed since age three, then take a trip to the playground or the supermarket. Later we'll share birthday cake and open his presents: an electric paper shredder and a toy keyboard. After his dinner—white rice with soy sauce, a few pieces of chicken, some grapes—he'll watch *Mary Poppins* for the five-hundredth time. In most respects, Cam's birthday will be just like every other summer day. And that's exactly how he wants it.

Cameron has autism, and for him our everyday world is a chaotic whirl: noises inaudible or innocuous to us drive him crazy; shadows and strings constantly distract him; words break up like radio signals drowned out by static. Any change in his routine makes Cam anxious, so my wife Leslie and I reshape our world in his image—visiting the same places, serving him the same foods, playing the same videos and CDs. In his world, a few insignificant objects become essential, as if imbued with magical properties, while objects significant to other people carry no meaning for him at all.

But Leslie and I also inhabit the "normal" world, so dwelling in Cameron's world is difficult. We can't always tell what he wants and often can't make him understand us; we feel oppressed by his rigid routines and his inability to learn. We are saddened by his chronic pain, the result of trying to fit into a world not made for him. Because the neuro-typical world demands that Cam live in it, he clings to those magical objects that cradle him in their consoling captivity.

Here is how life works in Cam's world.

He is fascinated by plants. But his botanical interest is less a scientist's than a locust's: he spends hours stripping the leaves from bushes and trees. Full of trees and rimmed by a forsythia hedge, our yard provides plenty of raw material, and, if left to his own devices, he'd denude it within days. If we look away for a moment, we'll find him three yards over, pulling leaves from a neighbor's dogwoods.

And so after lunch on his birthday, we visit a nearby playground, where at least he won't trespass or damage a neighbor's prize flowers. For us, the word "playground" is somewhat of a misnomer: Cam doesn't really play. In his eyes, the playground is simply a space full of plants helpfully arrayed for destruction. He roams, breaking branches from bushes or saplings. After snapping off a twig with his right hand, he runs his left hand along its length, briskly cleaning the limb. He repeats the action over and over, relentlessly. After husking the handiest bushes around the perimeter, he hops on the swings for a few minutes, as if to catch his breath, then returns to his botanical operations.

Why does he destroy plants? The professionals call these behaviors "self-stimulation," or "stims," or "stereotypies." It's as if an endless loop in Cam's brain places him on a treadmill he can neither shut off nor jump off. Yet his actions aren't just automatic: if you watch closely, you see that he carefully selects which stems to pull, having learned which plants have barbs or thorns, which are woody or limp, and which offer the precise degree of desirable resistance. Beyond these choices, however, each action is a near-perfect copy of the previous one. His work yields a purified present, a limbo where he can live more comfortably.

Above us, on the ball field, a father pitches softballs to a boy about Cam's age. The father maintains a stream of encouraging patter, coaching the boy to stay back and keep his eye on the ball, reminding him, "If you hit, run! Don't wait to see where it went."

I sit on a bench with a book while Cam strolls around stripping twigs. Then I saunter over and talk to him about the plants, naming each one as we walk. Am I putting on a show for the other father, pretending that this is an educational outing? Do I really think Cam understands or will remember what I say? Do I feel guilty for allowing him to peel trees? Or am I trying to salvage a sliver of the kind of father-son interaction I witness nearby? While the other dad teaches his son a sport, I'm just killing time, waiting for the dinner hour, waiting for the next day, which will be the same as this one—waiting for changes that never come.

Cam's unchanging world has become ours.

By the standards of our hybrid world, the playground outing is a success. But birthdays—so fraught with expectations—also expose the rift between Cam's standards and ours: we still find ourselves hoping he'll suddenly start acting like other kids. Our expectations make him anxious, so birthdays usually bring at least one serious tantrum: he may hit Leslie, tear my shirt to shreds, or try to bite one of us. We'll coax or wrestle him into his bedroom, or simply leave the room until he calms down.

But nothing like that happens today: we adjusted to his world instead of asking him to fit into ours. It's a happy birthday.

Temple Grandin, the highly intelligent autistic woman who has written books and been profiled by neurologist Oliver Sacks, describes feeling like an alien among neuro-typical people, comparing herself to an "anthropologist on Mars." Her description rings true, for each day with Cam shows us that although people like him and Grandin live in our world, they aren't truly *of* our world; they just drop in from time to time. And Cam sometimes seems to receive messages from that other world; when he does, he jams his fingers into his ears as if to block them out—or let his brain decipher them.

Last night Cam showed us again how he feels on our planet.

Movies generally baffle him: he can't make sense of the story and finds the characters' interactions unfathomable or boring. But last evening Leslie persuaded him to watch *The Wizard of Oz* with her. She explained the plot in simple terms as Dorothy sang "Over the Rainbow," got swept up in the cyclone, accidentally killed the Wicked Witch, met the singing Munchkins, collected the Scarecrow, Tin Man, and Cowardly Lion, and followed the Yellow Brick Road to seek the wonderful Wizard of Oz.

Cam perked up during the cyclone and songs, but grew restless during the dialogue sections. From the next room I heard mounting protests: loud claps, growls, vehement reiterations of "huh-uh-huh-uh-huh-uh." Then he prowled the house, pulling strings from the carpet, running water into the sink, slapping the walls.

After an hour of this, we put him to bed, but he couldn't sleep. Had the movie upset him? He'd just returned from his first stay at overnight camp, so maybe the story of a child whisked from home to a beautiful, frightening place reminded him of his own recent experiences. At camp, he too had been introduced to unusual creatures (in his case, horses) and to strangers small and large. When a thunderstorm struck that evening, did he fear it would pick up the house and fling him into Oz?

"There's no place like home," Dorothy chants, then awakes in her own bed. For Cam, the tale's most terrifying aspect may be that home often feels like Oz. There's no waking up for him.

How uncanny it is to recall the day exactly eleven years earlier when Leslie and I woke to find ourselves transported to a strange land from which we have never returned.

Part One

Awakenings

Chapter 1

Yankee Doodle Dandy

They enter the new world naked,
cold, uncertain of all
save that they enter . . .
—William Carlos Williams, "Spring and All"

Two of Us

July 4, 1989, dawned drearily: a cold, rainy day sure to dampen fireworks and drown high spirits. But Les and I weren't aware of the weather when she woke at 6 a.m. complaining of stomach pain.

"You need to get up, Wallace," she said. This nickname evolved from our habit of calling each other "Watson": we were each Holmes, addressing the other as his faithful, somewhat dim assistant. "Watson" became "Wats," and eventually, through Leslie's penchant for wordplay, "Wallace."

"Mmm. What's the matter?"

"I just bled into the toilet. I think I might be in labor. But something's wrong. I don't think I'm supposed to be bleeding."

"Is it just 'spotting'?"

"I don't think so. That was over months ago."

"Does it hurt a lot?"

"Not that much."

"Well, then, let's go back to sleep and deal with it when we get up." This couldn't be labor. She was only thirty-four weeks along and we didn't even have a crib yet. I rolled over to catch more winks.

Not reassured, my wife phoned her obstetrician, who was fortunately on call. "This isn't good," she said. "You need to go to St. Giles right away. I'll meet you there."

Then I started to worry.

We threw some toiletries into a bag and jumped into our rusting 1980 Toyota. Luckily, York Road, one of Baltimore's main drags, was almost deserted on the rainy holiday morning, and I hit 60 miles per hour crossing a usually busy intersection. Les was silent for most of the trip, her face turning paler by the minute.

After we checked in, a short, bespectacled woman entered our semiprivate room: the obstetrician, Dr. Zollar.

Upon examining my wife, the doctor said, "I think you've had a placental abruption. That means that the placenta has torn away from the wall of the uterus, which accounts for the bleeding. We can't let it go on long, because the baby could be losing blood. Your body wants to go into labor, but the birth canal isn't cooperating. So I'm going to give you this drug to induce labor."

As we waited for the drug to work, I recalled a silly argument from the night before. Les had insisted that we eat Kentucky Fried Chicken, which I can't stomach. There was no KFC near our rented house. I wasn't the most accommodating husband. Okay, I was rigid. As we trolled for chicken, I grew impatient.

"Why does it have to be Kentucky Fried? All that grease gives me heartburn."

"I just have this craving. Please, just this one time." She tightened her lips. I knew the look: she was very angry and pretending not to be, or had made up her mind to *get* angry if I persisted. "You could be more thoughtful, since I'm pregnant with *our* child."

"God, I'm sick of these cravings. If you don't want to cook, why don't we just order pizza?"

"You can never just give in, can you?" Her voice had acquired an edge. We were now moving onto the well-traveled terrain of my inflexibility.

"Relax! I'm giving in, for Christ's sake!" We finally located a KFC in a seedy neighborhood, then drove home in sullen silence. We grimly chewed the chicken parts, licking our wounds along with our fingers.

The next morning this conflict seemed trivial.

The nurse regularly checked for dilation. At 10 a.m., the doctor examined Leslie again and outlined our choices.

"This isn't working. We can continue to wait, and there's a possibility that the bleeding will stop or the drugs will start working. But I'm worried that the baby is losing blood. The conservative choice is to wait and see, but I recommend we go ahead and take the child."

"'Take.' You mean have the baby now?"

"That's right."

The two of us looked at each other and swallowed. This was happening much too fast.

At 10:45, Les was in the prep room phoning her mother. The doctor administered a spinal anesthetic, and by 11 I sat in scrubs watching the doctor perform a C-section. Les and I were conscious but dazed. We'd planned so meticulously: the weeks of Lamaze classes, puffing and panting beside other anxious parents-to-be; the careful modifications of the second bedroom; the giddy shopping for baby clothes. A premature birth was not in the plan!

I tried to stay chipper, but the doctor acted as though I'd faint any moment. Les kept asking, "Am I doing okay, Wall?"

"You're doing great, sweetie," I said, wiping my clammy hands.

As I numbly watched the procedure, Dr. Zollar glanced up and remarked, "In college, Wallace Stevens was my favorite poet."

"Yes, I like him very much too." What in hell was she talking about? Had I told her I was an English professor? And anyway, shouldn't we be discussing William Carlos Williams—the baby doctor? Then I realized that she thought my name was Wallace; that was what Leslie had been calling me since we'd arrived.

Moments later the doctor held up a slimy, wailing, reddish creature for our admiration. "A little boy!" she said. I could barely see him: my glasses had fogged up. A nurse cleaned off our son and handed him to Leslie. I wept quietly.

"You can hold him for a moment, but we have to get him to ICU right away," the nurse cautioned.

I called my parents, then sat with Les in post-op. Within minutes she was groaning in pain as her uterus contracted. When we'd first entered the room, we'd been surrounded by people. Now, suddenly, the place was deserted. Leslie's moans grew louder as her face turned gray.

Panicked, I raced to the nurses' station.

"My wife is in severe pain here! Can't you people do something!?"

The OB nurses, accustomed to dazzled new mothers and distraught new dads, treated us with crisp compassion, reassuring Leslie, administering another anesthetic, patting me on the shoulder. At last Les's pain abated, and we were sent to a private room. Once she fell asleep, I drove home to get clothes and toiletries.

The house was uncannily unchanged. There was the sock I'd dropped on the floor the night before, and here was the half-read copy of *Premiere,* still folded down to the Dustin Hoffman article, tossed negligently on the couch. The place looked as if we'd just stepped out for a lengthy breakfast. How could these small things still be the same when we'd just been hit by a tornado?

I fed our calico cat and scratched her ears. "You don't know it, Vida, but you're about to be ousted from the number one spot." She purred contentedly in my lap.

As I caught my breath, I recalled the circuitous journey that had brought us from our shared home ground, a tiny logging town in northwestern Montana, to a big eastern city.

Not long after we married in 1981, we caught a lucky break: I won a fellowship (funded, in a coincidence that still prompts chuckles, by Coca-Cola, Cam's favorite beverage) to enter the PhD program at Emory University in Atlanta. Off we went—reverse pioneers, hicks from the sticks venturing east to test our mettle.

When I landed a teaching job in Baltimore, we threw away the birth control. The pregnancy months were blissful, and we grew exhilarated at the idea of having a baby. Aside from a bout of what seemed to be food poisoning during a visit with relatives in Seattle, Les had been free from illness.

Despite our occasional bickering, the pregnancy had strengthened our bond, and it's a good thing it did, for we really had nobody else. That's what struck me hardest as I gazed around the house: we were all alone here. Our families were thousands of miles away, back in Montana. And even if they had lived near us, they were consumed with their own problems: our fathers' failing businesses, my father's new family, Les's brother's illness. Moving east had let us jettison this baggage and start over.

Nevertheless, we still thought like Westerners: we believed we could overcome any obstacle with toughness and hard work. Alone again in a huge, unfamiliar city, we adopted the Beatles' "Two of Us" as our song: we were the lovers "wearing raincoats / standing solo in the sun." We trusted each other totally and needed no one else.

As I sat in the empty house, our independence seemed foolhardy. If something bad happened, we had nobody to bail us out. My stomach roiled as I imagined my wife dying, the baby blind or disabled. But I quickly banished these thoughts. There were things to be done: return to the hospital, stay with Les, and tomorrow get busy fixing up the baby's room.

We tried to get used to the idea that we'd become parents. But I was still rattled and told everyone who happened by that our baby was five weeks early. "We don't even have a crib," I announced to every stranger.

The next morning we visited our son—a tiny, wrinkled specimen of humanity surrounded by IV lines and lying in an incubator. He looked an awful lot like a monkey. I still have the birth photo: it's nearly impossible to recognize our dark-haired, dark-eyed boy in this skinny, rubicund little thing. He looks like a miniature, slightly botched, clay copy of me.

We named him Cameron Scott. His middle name honored Leslie's youngest brother, who'd recently undergone a kidney transplant.

A superstitious person might have viewed the name as a bad omen.

Three of Us

Cam had trouble breathing on his own; he was jaundiced, underweight and generally looked half-baked. But at 5 pounds, 3 ounces, he was a linebacker compared to the other infants in the ward. I remember staring with amazement at one wee girl with a head about the size of a large plum. She weighed a pound and a half. How could a human being be so minute?

Our baby looked as if he'd shatter with a single touch. I could hardly bear to look at him for even a few minutes. Whenever he stopped breathing for a second, my own would halt as well. I desperately wanted to hold him, talk to him, tell him my plans and dreams. At the same time, I was afraid that I'd do irreparable harm if I so much as patted his tiny head. I thought of him as a foundling from another planet who couldn't adjust to our atmosphere and had to wear a space suit.

"E. T., phone home," I whispered through the glass.

For brief periods after feeding, I was allowed to hold him in my arms. Cradling him, I'd softly sing:

> I'm a Yankee Doodle dandy,
> A Yankee Doodle do or die!
> A real-live nephew of my Uncle Scott
> Born on the Fourth of July.

Les was determined that our dandy would start life the right way. She couldn't breastfeed him in ICU—he couldn't nurse on his own yet, anyway—so several times a day she borrowed the hospital breast pump and filled bottles with her milk. This gadget was more precious than rubies, and every few hours we'd have to enlist a nurse to find which new mom was hoarding the pump. After a couple of days, I went to buy one for ourselves alone.

I roamed the Rite-Aid, screwing up the courage to talk to the sales clerk. At last I strode up and said in my most insouciant voice, "I'm looking for a breast pump."

She looked quizzically at my chest. "Right over here, sir. What size?"

"Um, large, I guess," I stammered, staring down at my sneakers.

Parenthood was a brave new world, all right. But Les was equal to it: unlike the other mothers, still bedridden several days following their deliveries, she began walking around the day after her C-section. We happily cooked up plans for our son.

"Cameron. Do you think that sounds like a lawyer's name?" she asked.

"More like an actor."

"C. S. Osteen. What about a writer?"

"Or a scholar."

"Nah. One of those is enough. Somebody will have to take care of us when we get old."

"I hope he has your looks."

"Oh, Wallace." She smiled brightly. "I hope he has your brain and voice."

"There's nothing wrong with your brain, hon. But please God, spare him these eyes," I said, turning mine up toward heaven and removing my thick glasses.

After five days, Leslie came home. The experience felt surreal: we'd gone to the hospital, where she'd left a child. Then we came back without him. Did we really have a baby, or was this some vivid dream that was now dissolving? If so, how could we explain those bottles of milk lined up in the fridge like little white soldiers?

We lived in limbo. Several times a day we'd go to the hospital, feed and cuddle our child, wait until he fell asleep, then put him back in his crib and return home. The place had never seemed so empty.

We had a new baby, and yet we didn't.

Finally, on the twelfth day, after Cam began to put on weight, the doctors let us take him home. I'd bought a new car seat for him, only to discover that the lap belts of our old Corolla had rusted into the latches. You couldn't pull them out with a winch. The nearest junkyards were miles away and I simply didn't have the energy to canvass them.

So we brought our new baby directly from the hospital to the auto dealer, and that day purchased our first new car, a silver Toyota Corolla we named Sam. Its key feature: working seat belts. Sam and Cam came home the same day— July 16, 1989.

Leaving the dealership, we sang a chorus of "Two of Us," forgetting that the title no longer fit. No matter: we were on our way home!

With a new boy and a new car, our happiness seemed complete. Yet we still hadn't completely adjusted to the new situation. A week or so later, realizing we had nothing for dinner, Les and I trotted out to the car to make a grocery run. As I turned the key I looked at her.

"Are we forgetting something?"

"Oh my God! The baby!" We burst out laughing, then quickly sobered at the realization that a little being now depended on us completely. A profound change had come upon us: for the first time we grasped the enormous responsibility we'd assumed. We couldn't move away from this one: Cam was a lifetime commitment.

The next year was the happiest of our lives. Cameron quickly fattened up on his mother's milk, and by the end of the year was in the fiftieth percentile for his age. He was a quiet, happy baby. After ten weeks, we placed him in a home-based day care with Maggie Schubert, a gentle, experienced woman in her forties who had tended dozens of infants and thought Cam was beautiful. Les returned to work in her home office.

Cameron hit a couple of milestones a little late, but we chalked it up to prematurity and didn't worry much. He was a gregarious baby who smiled and clapped at everyone he saw. His first word—at ten months of age—was "Hi." In fact, he spoke before he walked.

He was precocious in other respects as well. Before he was a year old, we had purchased a whole library of toddler books: *Where Is Spot?*, *Max's Bath*, *Bear Goes Shopping*, *Goodnight, Moon*. He wanted to "read" these books constantly and before long had them all memorized.

At twelve months old, Cam was just taking his first steps; our move to a new house set him back a few weeks, but he was walking on his own soon after his first birthday. His movements were unusual: he'd often stop in an odd position, one leg extended straight behind him, as if he'd suddenly forgotten where it was supposed to go. And he never really toddled; as soon as he was able to walk, he wanted to run. But we were far too consumed with furnishing our new house, consoling our disgruntled cat, and caring for our child to notice anything out of the ordinary—if anything was.

I have a photo from this period displayed in my office: our one-year-old is turned to the left, smiling brightly as he stands near *Spot's Birthday Party*, holding a blue stacking cup. He poses in bright orange shorts and shirt before the uncurtained window of our new house, his face beaming out of the dark background. The world glistens with possibility.

Chapter 2

The News

From childhood's hour I have not been
As others were—I have not seen
As others saw—I could not bring
My passions from a common spring. . . .
—Edgar Allan Poe, "Alone"

The Prodigy

I scan a photo of Leslie and Cam sitting on the couch in our rental house. He couldn't be more than ten months old, yet here he is, lifting a flap in a *Spot* book to see what's beneath it. The concentration in his eyes is remarkable. Here is a similar photo of Cam at nine months, sitting on my lap, staring intently at the newspaper. You'd swear he is reading the headlines.

Toddler Cam was indeed unusual. He didn't reach out when he wanted to be picked up and seldom made the kind of eye contact that means "I'm looking at you and want you to look at me because I'm trying to tell you something." He didn't babble like most babies and, as a toddler, never played with toys, except by mouthing them.

Yet he loved his Johnny jump-up, a moveable swing we placed in the archways of our house. He'd happily bob and up and down for a half-hour at a stretch. If now this habit seems a precursor of autistic rocking, at the time it was just a good way to give him exercise and keep him occupied.

If we'd had other children, we might have been concerned about Cam's focus on books, which deepened as he entered his second year. If Les said, "Go get Spot," Cam would run to his bedroom and emerge with an oversized book clutched in his tiny hands, sometimes dropping it but determinedly dragging it to his mother, then crawl into her lap to hear the familiar stories. One of us would act out the voices in *Where's Spot?* He loved hearing us roar like a lion or assume the alligator's voice. He'd sit for hours at a time, reading book after book, or the same book over and over. By age two, he had several of them memorized.

We were thrilled by his prodigious interest. It was marvelous to see our son so captivated, to watch him try to grasp the concepts, to teach him to turn pages with his chubby fingers.

At his one-year checkup, we asked our pediatrician about his "reading" habit. We added that Cam didn't want to play with toys and ignored other kids. The doctor smiled indulgently, no doubt pigeonholing us as oversolicitous yuppie parents. But when Leslie mentioned to a neighbor, a pediatric nurse, that all Cam wanted to do was "read" books, the neighbor blanched. Later she confided that Cam's lack of interest in toys and obsession with books had raised a red flag.

But others we trusted noticed nothing amiss. On a visit with relatives in Seattle, my aunt and uncle, retired speech pathologists, told us that "everything was lined up" for Cam (then sixteen months old) to start talking. And when we traveled to Montana as Cam was turning two, my closest uncle watched our son pore over his books and predicted we had a prodigy on our hands. Cam *did* seem precocious; but if his concentration was extraordinary, it was also one-dimensional. Would he become a nerd who only wanted to stay in his room and read?

It was easy to reason that our boy was like his parents, whose love for reading had sustained us through our troubled childhoods. We thought his fascination was charming, especially since he wanted to "read" only to Leslie—as if Dad, with his PhD in English, wasn't qualified to read *Spot's Birthday Party*.

Then the Max books became Cam's favorites. He'd cue us to read *Max's Toys:*

Cam: Max wuv Ruby dah Emiwy . . . [Max loved Ruby's doll, Emily.]
Les: So much. "Max," said Ruby, "Emily is . . ."
Cam: One ting . . .
Les: . . . you may not have.

These little tales were soon permanently imprinted on our brains. They became our private family code.

Before long, Cam could recognize certain words—"ball," "cup," "run." If we'd been child development experts this hyperlexia would have worried us, since it often presages autism. Like many hyperlexic kids, Cam didn't connect the printed words with things in the outside world, nor understand the ideas involved: he loved the Spot book called *Opposites,* yet didn't grasp the concept of opposition. Nor did he realize that he was supposed to guess what Bear in *Bear Goes Shopping* would wear or buy based on the season or store. He couldn't point to the correct answer; in fact, he didn't seem to understand that a question was being asked. And he had no desire to show us anything.

By age three, Cam's interest in books was waning. By age five, he'd barely look at them. Could we have taken more advantage of this savant-like skill? Would doing so have made a difference? We don't know. But over the years, Cam's loss of interest in reading became for us a symbol of his autism, an emblem of lost opportunity: first he could read, and then he couldn't.

The Strangers

In our new-parent bliss, we saw only the bright, cheerful little guy displayed in a photo we took just before Christmas 1990: smiling broadly, Cameron seems perfectly at home in the world. His next photo, taken in March, shows a slightly different child. He is clapping, but his smile looks slightly askew, his eyes unfocused. At the earlier session, he'd been tractable and calm; at the second, he was cranky and restless. He wouldn't pose and couldn't sit still. This photo captures for me the moment when things began to go wrong, when our first lives as parents of a bright, promising boy gave way to our second lives as parents of a disabled child.

More troubling: he no longer said "hi," never said "mommy," and couldn't put two words together. His fine motor skills hadn't advanced beyond grasping objects with his entire hand. Most bewildering of all: he didn't respond to his own name.

We began to suspect that he was developmentally delayed. But these fears didn't coalesce until the spring of 1991. That's when Cam began bawling inconsolably and throwing himself on the floor at Maggie's day care every time another parent came to drop off or pick up a child. It was as if he couldn't distinguish his parents from other adults. These fits seemed out of character for our busy but affable child. Maggie tried picking him up when he cried; she tried ignoring the tantrums; she tried putting him in a room by himself. Nothing helped. He stopped wailing only when he wore himself out.

We tried to write it off as a typical two-year-old's stranger anxiety, but Maggie was concerned. Day after day, Les or I would pick up our traumatized toddler only to be regaled with another story of his inexplicable and (she made it clear) appalling behavior. Afterward, I'd take Cam to the playground near our house. He'd run back and forth on the empty basketball courts, following the painted lines as if obeying some private rule. The exercise gave relief to him, but not to us, for it was clear that something frightening was unfolding.

One day I arrived at day care and found Cameron in the throes of a huge tantrum. Maggie's adult daughter, who'd been watching Cam that day, told us she'd been "firm" with him when he'd thrown something on the floor. The next day, he screamed every time she entered the room. Our first thought was the same as any parent's: she had harmed him. Now we had a straw to grasp—maybe we could chalk up his tantrums to maltreatment.

We described Cam's behavior to our pediatrician, who also raised the possibility of molestation. But it was hard to concentrate on his words because Cam was having one of the screaming panic attacks that had become regular occurrences whenever we entered his waiting room. The other kids would stare, and their parents would give us a look that said, "I wouldn't let *my* child get away with this." We felt utterly inadequate.

By midsummer, we'd removed Cam from day care, still clinging to the belief that someone had hurt or frightened him. How else to explain his profound, seemingly unmotivated terror? We soldiered on, hoping his problems would cure themselves or vanish as mysteriously as they'd appeared. Fortunately Les worked at home, and since I didn't teach during the summer, we could share child-care duties.

But tantrums were no longer our only concern. Encounters with other children made it increasingly obvious that something wasn't right with our son.

When a neighbor boy about Cam's age had visited us the previous winter, we'd noted proudly that our son spoke more clearly, ran faster, and followed directions better than the other boy. A dinner party with that family a few months later revealed that the other boy had passed Cam by. We adults sat in lawn chairs while the guests' two sons raced around exploring. Cam's peer chased the fireflies flitting across the yard. "Look!" he shouted, racing after them, trying to snatch one in his hand. "Look at that!" he yelled, pointing.

Cam paid no attention to the boys. In the deepening dusk I grabbed his hand and trailed after them, trying to direct his gaze to the illuminated insects. But he didn't try to catch them; he didn't seem to *see* them. He didn't even seem to understand what "look" meant. I pretended he was being bratty but knew in my heart that something was wrong. Why wouldn't he look up? Was he nearsighted or partially blind? And why wouldn't he come when we called his name? Was he just ignoring us, or did he not understand what we were saying?

By Halloween, our house was a horror chamber, but not because of scary costumes. At every ring of the doorbell, Cameron fled shrieking or dropped to the floor in a paroxysm of fear. We handed out candy to the costumed kids, ignoring our child's demonic cries. What was he afraid of? What did he want?

Our son's world was filled with foes and strangers. And as autism hijacked his development, he became more and more a stranger to us.

The Experts

If we'd known more about child development, it would have been obvious what was occurring. Setbacks in language development at about eighteen months, no interest in toys or interaction with others: Cameron was exhibiting the textbook signs of autism.

But our pediatrician was also ignorant. At our next appointment, he gave us a book called *The Difficult Child,* explaining that some kids get stubborn and uncontrollable between ages two and three. We were tremendously relieved: this was just an exaggerated case of the terrible twos! We read the book, recognizing some of Cam's troublesome behaviors. I remembered that my sister had been a difficult toddler but then became a friendly, though moody, child. Perhaps things weren't so dire after all.

Cam began to watch himself obsessively in our living room's large mirror. His actions seemed both unfocused and charged with unquellable anxiety: he couldn't sit still but couldn't do anything meaningful, either. He greeted our efforts to interest him in Legos and Elmo dolls with indifference or hostility. Even *Where's Spot?* had lost its charm.

To provide an outlet for his brimming energy, we bought a small exercise trampoline and placed it in front of the living room window. Cam soon became strongly attached to the tramp, jumping on it before, during, and after other activities, usually while watching himself in the mirror. "Loo-ee, loo-ee," he'd declare, bouncing, springing off and running away, then returning to bounce some more.

With Les still working at home, we got by. The days were stressful: I was trying to earn tenure and Les's boss suspected that she really wasn't working. But we still wrote off Cam's odd behaviors as eccentricity or delay. Our pediatrician wasn't alarmed, so why should we be?

Then, one afternoon in the fall of 1991, Les arrived home looking pale and frightened. While browsing in the child-care section of a local bookstore, she had stumbled upon *Children with Autism: A Parent's Guide,* an introduction to the disorder containing quotations from parents about their autistic children's behaviors.

"Wallace, I saw this book in the bookstore that describes Cam. Bunny, I think this is it. I'm afraid even to say this, but I think Cam might be autistic."

"Autistic! I doubt it!" I frowned. "That's really rare. Anyway, isn't lack of eye contact one of the main signs? You know he makes eye contact with us."

"No, he doesn't, not really. They also mention that these kids make weird finger motions. Yesterday I saw him flap his fingers while he looked at himself in the mirror." She was on the verge of tears.

"Oh, he's just waving at himself," I told her.

"You can deny it if you want to, but this book explains what autistic kids are like and Cam sounds just like them. It's like somebody hit me over the head with a club. This is it, I know it. This is what's wrong with him."

I wasn't denying what I secretly knew; I actually wasn't worried. All I knew about autism came from the movie *Rain Man* and Oliver Sacks's *The Man Who Mistook His Wife for a Hat.* I didn't connect Cam's reading obsession with these characters' eccentricities. Besides, autism was so rare—might as well worry about being struck by lightning!

Les insisted that I read the book, and I had to admit that the kids in some of the stories resembled Cam. But what *was* autism? Were there any therapies for it? Did kids get over it?

At our next appointment, we pushed our pediatrician to acknowledge Cam's delayed development. Although it should have been obvious from the raging tantrums he'd witnessed that our child was excessively anxious, he still rolled his eyes whenever our son screamed, and gave the impression we were letting him get away with murder. But at least he provided the name and number of a Baltimore County agency that targeted developmentally delayed toddlers and infants. Leslie made the appointment.

In the meantime, we'd found another day care only three blocks from our house. Make Room for Darlings was operated by Ms. Helga, a heavy, gray-haired woman with a German accent. She seemed a bit rigid, but the place featured a large jungle gym and looked clean and well-run, so we decided to send Cam there for half-days. If something bad happened, we could be at her door within two minutes.

Helga conformed all too well to the stereotype of the dictatorial Teuton. The kids had to line up for everything and put their toys away after each play session (these were two- and three-year-olds). Fitting in was paramount; Cam didn't fit in.

One day Helga pulled me aside and asked, "Does he have to put away his toys at home?"

He didn't play with toys, so he hardly needed to put them away. I shook my head.

Her mouth was a pinched line. "He won't follow directions. He seems completely unsocialized." Her meaning was crystal clear: Cam's main problem was his lousy parents. In her considered opinion, he was spoiled rotten. The accusation annoyed us, but Cam seemed to enjoy going there, so we stuck with it.

A couple of months later, he fell from her jungle gym and knocked loose a front tooth, requiring a visit to the dentist. Fortunately, there was no serious damage. The next day Helga explained that Cam had fallen while climbing the ladder up to the slide. I wasn't sure whether to blame her or apologize for my uncoordinated son. I laughed it off, but she seemed worried. We didn't know it, but Cam's placement was shakier than his tooth.

March 26, 1992, was the date of our assessment with LOCATE, the county agency. It was the day we first glimpsed our future. Nearby Red Willow School was the evaluation site. There we met Rhonda Hart, a woman of about forty-five with warm blue eyes and a comforting manner: a charming combination of laid-back, aging hippie and wealthy matron.

Hart and a speech pathologist tried to get Cam to play ball, evaluated his verbal comprehension, and tested his motor skills with keys and screw tops. Right away they began exchanging cryptic remarks: "Is that real laughter or just self-stim?" "He doesn't seem to notice that we're talking to him." "See any shared attention?" They also asked us questions: does he point to things for you to look at? Does he follow directions? Leslie told them Cam's linguistic abilities had declined between fourteen and twenty months and that he didn't play with toys.

Although they suggested that he was developmentally delayed, their demeanor was reassuring. Their written evaluation was not: "Cameron mouthed objects and did not like to be touched; . . . he randomly explored toys yet did not use them appropriately; he did not follow verbal directions. . . . He vocalized a laugh sound which may be a self-stimulatory utterance. . . . He did not use any words during the evaluation."

These professionals knew what was wrong, yet never once uttered the word "autism." In fact, when Les asked Ms. Hart straight out if Cameron was autistic, she said, "We prefer not to use labels." A few minutes later she whispered to Leslie, "I think it's PDD."

"What's that?"

"Pervasive developmental disorder. It means he has some developmental delays that we can't nail down exactly."

The word "pervasive" sounded ominous, but not as scary as "autism." Even so, their evaluation frightened us. At thirty-three months of age, Cam's play skills and verbal pragmatics (that is, his ability to use words to communicate and affect others) stood at the twelve- to eighteen-month level. His language comprehension and expression were that of a sixteen-month-old. His perceptual fine motor skills, cognition, and social-emotional abilities were all between twelve- and twenty-month levels. In short, Cam was half as far along as most kids his age. They recommended that he receive speech/language services and enroll in the parent/infant program to "stimulate receptive and expressive language development."

I tried to shrug off the assessment by fixing on minute disagreements between the evaluators. Wasn't he learning to jump? Wasn't he starting to walk up stairs? Couldn't he recite entire books? On a deeper level, I may have known I was kidding myself. But accepting that my son might be autistic or otherwise disabled would mean that we'd failed almost before we'd begun. It would mean that my son was a stranger, someone quite unlike me or my wife—or just about anybody else we knew.

The evaluation was gratifying to one person: Ms. Helga. The next day, she asked me about the assessment.

"They told us he's delayed in almost every area. I think they exaggerated a little. But we're going to work really hard and get him caught up."

She looked dubious. "What did they say about his behavior?"

"They said it was part of his delay. He doesn't understand language very well and that's why he can't follow directions."

She sniffed. "He just doesn't listen. He is off by himself and doesn't play with the other children. And he breaks things. He's very destructive." She didn't need experts to tell her what she already knew: Cameron was a *bad boy*—certainly not one of her kind.

Voyagers

In April 1992, we told Rhonda we were planning to visit Ireland for ten days so I could attend a James Joyce conference. She laughed incredulously.

"You're going to Ireland with a PDD kid!" she exclaimed. "I'm not sure whether you're brave or foolish."

We were too ignorant to know the risks we were taking. The voyage was uneventful—aside from a sweltering two-hour wait on the tarmac at Shannon—until we finally deplaned in Dublin. At that point, Cam launched into a screaming, thrashing tantrum.

We shared a cab with a fellow Joyce scholar we'd encountered at baggage claim. Our son screamed as the four of us sat shoulder-to-armpit in the tiny cab, careening through Dublin's glistening, early-morning streets. The man sympathetically recalled trying to nap next to his daughter when she was Cam's age.

"It was like trying to sleep in a clothes dryer!" We all laughed. But by the time we arrived at the hotel a half-hour later, our good humor had vanished. When we tried to check in, the clerk informed us that our room wasn't ready. Leslie had had enough.

"Look," she said, "Either you get a room ready for us *now* or we're leaving this child down here with you while we find another hotel!"

The stammering desk clerk stared in horror at our squirming, shrieking kid, then immediately called the bellman. Within two minutes we were ensconced in a cramped room. Ten minutes later all three of us were sound asleep.

The rest of the trip went surprisingly well. While I attended sessions, Les took Cam for long walks through the city in his beloved stroller.

On the final day of the conference, we met on a grassy square at Trinity College where other families waited to see a Book of Kells exhibit. Freed from the stroller, Cam ran wild, climbing and tumbling all over the benches and stairs. After one ascent, he looked proudly up at his dad and announced, "Me!"

A nearby father herding his three rambunctious preschoolers glanced at me and said, with dry Irish humor, "That sums it all up for him, eh?"

"Yeah, he's the center of his world."

"Watch out. Next it will be 'Mine!'" I wish he'd been right.

After the conference, we drove a rented Ford through the western counties. Cameron sat calmly in his car seat as we hurtled down the narrow Irish highways from tourist site to tourist site. Afraid to risk dining in restaurants, we survived on peanut butter sandwiches and fruit; in our hotel rooms, we used the tea or coffee maker to heat water and make Cam's beloved oatmeal. Sated by room service dinners and soothed by abundant pints of Harp, we managed to enjoy ourselves.

The good times ended when we entered Shannon Airport for the return flight; Cameron immediately began screaming. He rolled, he rocked, he stamped his feet, his face went dark red. As soon as we exited the terminal, he quieted down. A few minutes later we went back inside, and when the next flight was announced, Cam started to scream again. Then we got it: the PA system was pitched in a register he couldn't stand. For the first time, we realized that Cam's hearing was not like other people's, that certain sounds—innocuous to us— hurt his ears.

The flight back was a mélange of crunched pretzels, puddles of apple juice, and smelly diapers. After landing at Boston's packed Logan Airport during a hot afternoon rush hour, we had to take a bus to the terminal where we'd catch our flight to Baltimore. Already near the breaking point when we landed, Cam commenced wailing after a few seconds on the crowded bus. Our fellow passengers, mostly middle-aged businessmen, treated us compassionately. No doubt we looked pitiful: jet-lagged voyagers lugging a squalling kid.

"Long day, huh?" remarked a man in a gray suit.

"My kid gets like that every afternoon," another said.

"You guys hang in there," one businessman said. "He'll get over it."

Back in Baltimore, our house reeked of cat vomit. Vida, the twelve-year-old calico who'd been with us since those long-ago days in Montana, had been ill before we'd left, and now couldn't keep down any food. Patches of dark, tarry vomit decorated the floor and couch. The stains on the rug and sofa seemed to rebuke us: how dare we travel the world when our cat was sick and our child had a developmental disorder?

The next Monday, Les drove Cam to Make Room for Darlings but returned five minutes later. "She wouldn't let him come back," she gasped out. The story emerged between sobs.

Helga had placed her stout body in the threshold. "You may not bring him in. He can't come back to my day care. He's not like the other kids. I can't do anything with him." She was valiantly protecting her children from a monster or contagion.

She had no room for our darling.

As Les turned to leave, Helga had relented slightly. "He can visit from time to time. If he starts doing better, maybe he can come back." Fat chance. We wouldn't have gone back there if she ran the only day care in Baltimore.

The "A" Word

When I studied the developmental chart in Powers's book, I saw that Cam was clearly delayed—but not in every category. I was certain that he knew more than ten words and that he could feed himself almost without help (a thirty-six-month milestone). His stranger anxiety was abating, he had fewer tantrums and slept well, and the folks at LOCATE seemed optimistic.

I didn't want Cam to be autistic, so he wasn't.

But not long after our return from Ireland, Les went to Red Willow School to discuss a hearing test with an audiologist. As soon as she described Cam's symptoms, the audiologist said, "You should go back to your pediatrician and ask for a thorough examination. What you've described sounds to me like infantile autism."

That was the first time any professional had used the "A" word to refer to Cam.

The more we read about autism and the more we observed our son, the more we believed the audiologist's diagnosis. But when we returned to our pediatrician and told him that the LOCATE folks believed Cam had PDD or autism, his response was right out of a bad novel—his mouth actually fell open. He bustled around the office and made a big production out of photocopying the DSM-III description of "Pervasive Developmental Disorder."

Leslie asked about Cam's prognosis. "This isn't a death sentence," Tolbert answered. "He'll continue to grow and learn."

We jeered on the drive home. "Thanks for all your help, you little twink! Could you believe he actually showed us the DSM description?"

"That's probably all he knows about it!"

"At least now he doesn't think Cam's just spoiled."

By that evening, however, his feeble reassurance had begun to seem ominous: in his mind, the only thing worse than what Cam had was a terminal illness. His words spurred us on. We'd show him: we'd make Cam get better no matter *what* it took.

Chapter 3

Jabberwocky

Beware the jabberwock, my son!
The jaws that bite, the claws that catch!
—Lewis Carroll, *Through the Looking-Glass*

Faulty Switches

We began telling friends about Cam's disorder. "His brain is like an appliance that lacks an 'on' switch," I'd say. "We just have to bypass all the nonfunctional switches and turn everything on by hand. So instead of teaching the concept and then applying it, he'll have to learn everything by rote. But as soon as we get everything turned on, he should be running fine."

My metaphor was faulty, but it made me feel better. I was trying to describe a phenomenon I'd recently learned about—"weak central coherence." This is the theory that autistic people's skills are disconnected from each other, which makes it difficult for them to generalize from individual skills. Discrete trial therapy works by repeating drills until the child memorizes the skills and either grasps the principle or makes it unnecessary.

Under Rhonda Hart's guidance, we worked with Cam diligently every night for as long as he (and we) could stand it—about half an hour. We tried to teach him to pound different-sized pegs into a bench with a toy hammer, but he couldn't distinguish one shape from another or hang onto the hammer. Nor could he sit at the table for more than thirty seconds at a stretch, or point to a picture and tell what it was. In fact, he couldn't point, period.

We bought a toy parking garage, a play house, a tea set, a series of stuffed animals. Cam showed no interest in any of them. We laboriously tried to engage him in "let's pretend" games, to teach him to use the Busy Box, the See 'n' Say. Hand over hand, day after day, we'd pull down the lever and coax him to predict what came next, or make any choice at all. He eventually did learn to pull down the handle, but never linked the picture with the sounds. Not only didn't Cam know how to play; he didn't seem to want to.

We'd end each session with a singing game such as "Eensy Weensy Spider," or "She'll Be Comin' Round the Mountain." Les and I would loudly sing and urge Cam to join in, model the gestures, and place our hands over his. But all incoming transmissions were garbled: "the eensy weensy spider" got squashed into "eeen. . . . IDER"; "Comin' round the mountain" came out as "ountn . . . OMES." The next time, different syllables might be scrambled. Given his perceptual inconstancy, it's no wonder Cam couldn't sing along: he never heard the same song twice, and the words he did hear were gibberish.

We attempted to make the sessions enjoyable by laughing and jumping around. "This is fun!" we'd holler, but it wasn't fun for Les and me. Sweaty and frazzled, we'd emerge from Cam's room exhausted, not by our gymnastics but by the hard labor of trying to maintain his attention and by our growing frustration and feelings of helplessness.

Our praise didn't motivate him. What did work? After each session we went out for frozen yogurt. Aware that "i cree" was on the way, our fidgety, aimless child became focused and compliant. He used his spoon effectively and sometimes tossed the empty cup into the trash. So why couldn't he play a game or sing with us?

When it was time to show Rhonda what he'd learned at home, Cam would blank out, busy himself stacking chairs, and sneeze convulsively. At first I thought he was just stalling, but I soon came to believe he was responding to stress: these tasks were so hard for him that he got an "allergic" reaction when instructed to "do the puzzle," or "clap your hands like me!" But maybe his runny nose had a different cause—dust. Rhonda's office/playroom was cluttered with heaps of toys and learning aids—balls of all sizes, toy cash registers, cars and trucks, board games, puzzles, flash cards, dolls—and her desk and chair were buried beneath mounds of paper, books, and files.

Her methodology was similar: a random collection of ideas with no clear strategy. It seemed that she also lacked central coherence. One week we'd try interactive games; the next, problem solving; the next, word comprehension.

Then we'd return to something that had failed earlier. I couldn't decide whether she'd just forgotten (which was my suspicion) or wasn't letting us in on her master plan.

We were coming face-to-face with the meaning of "learning disability": the person can't acquire basic skills. It was becoming harder and harder to deny that Cam was cognitively impaired. What is intelligence if not the readiness to learn novel skills and the capacity to formulate plans and carry them out?

What did Cam like to do?

He loved to rock on a handmade wooden pony my mother had given him for his second Christmas. By age three he dwarfed the little pony but would still happily mount Old Paint, a huge smile pasted on his face, the big-eyed horse in an arrested prance: our own version of D. H. Lawrence's character in "The Rocking-Horse Winner" but without the luck. Cam's rocking troubled us, yet we couldn't bring ourselves to ban an activity he so enjoyed. Eventually we put Old Paint out to pasture, storing him in the crawl space where he still stares blankly into the darkness. Cam's rocking, however, never disappeared.

He also loved music. The anxious child beleaguered by a meaningless din became a tranquil lamb when listening to *Peter and the Wolf*. Upbeat tunes like "Knees Up, Mother Brown," or "John Jacob Jingleheimer Schmidt" prompted claps and shouts. Music was an island of order in a sea of chaos, a medium whose message, for some reason, arrived unscrambled. When music put the jabberwock to sleep in its cave, we glimpsed a calmer Cam.

He also loved to watch the videos we'd introduced at fourteen months old. He watched his Raffi concert videos every day—and I mean *every* day. I made a long dub tape of *Disney Singalong* and *Kidsongs* videos. For years, whenever Cam needed entertainment or consolation, we could switch on the videos and enjoy a brief respite. Good ol' black-bearded Raffi, with his guitar and sky-blue Hawaiian shirt, and friendly Scarecrow at Old McDonald's Farm: they were our constant companions. More than that, they were our saviors.

There were no surprises in Video World. The auditorium where Raffi sings, the farm where kids serenade a cow, the colorful land where Alice celebrates an unbirthday party, the village where Pinocchio trips over his own feet—these places were sensible and safe, unlike the real world, which buffeted Cam with unpredictable changes, incomprehensible chatter, and painful, overcharged sensations.

Back in this real world, our son spent hours making wave-like motions at the side of his face. It was as though the movements didn't originate in his own body, as if a short circuit permitted the message to flow from brain to fingers but blocked the returning message that announced, "This is your hand." Sometimes Cam seemed to fling imaginary water from his hands; other times he'd create fluttery shapes that transformed his otherwise maladroit fingers into magic butterflies. He seldom looked directly at his fingers, as if the shapes were too beautiful to bear when viewed straight on. Instead he gazed aslant, from the corner of his eyes.

But most of the time, he was a tiny dynamo whose relentless energy was diverted into meaningless (to us), repetitive activities. Our job wasn't really to turn on the switches but to direct his perpetual motion outward, into something meaningful.

Good Night Moon

We looked for a day care that would tolerate our unusual son. The women who ran these facilities displayed what we now called the Ms. Helga Syndrome: they were officious, rigid, moralistic. They'd never be able to cope with Cam. Three months after Helga had booted him out, we still hadn't found a replacement.

At last we discovered Good Night Moon, lodged in the second floor of a church in an older African-American neighborhood. It seemed our last chance. At our initial visit, we saw a toddler knock over a block pyramid and break into tears, but thirty seconds later a teacher had him giggling. We were impressed. But the main reason we sent Cam there was simpler: they accepted him.

Though Cam was now past three, he was placed with the two-year-olds taught by Miss Toni, a no-nonsense woman of about thirty-five. She kept a tight rein on her tykes, but beneath her tough exterior she was warm and loving. She didn't expect miracles; she just expected Cam to be his best self.

Miss T would gently coax him to participate in activities, but if he wanted to sit alone, wave his fingers and vocalize, she let him do it, at least briefly. "Cameron was talkin' to the angels again," she'd tell us later. Miss T was able to see, as few have since, that his autism is not only a disability but also a strange gift that sometimes tunes him to frequencies—the Wonderland frequency, maybe—the rest of us don't receive.

Good Night Moon made us believe that, in the right environment, Cam could thrive. But Red Willow's second assessment, in early 1993, darkened our horizon again. After nine months in their program, his skills remained at the twelve- to twenty-four-month level; he'd made virtually no progress. Yet the IEP (individual educational plan) they wrote a month later read, "the present placement is appropriate." Translation: they didn't expect much and couldn't do much for him.

We knew Cam needed something else but couldn't provide it ourselves. We both had demanding jobs, and Cam spent only mornings at Good Night Moon, which meant Leslie had to pick him up after lunch and then try to work—answering clients' calls, designing marketing strategies, discussing artwork—

while keeping our son occupied. On non-teaching days, I took over, but I was expected to prepare for class, attend meetings, and do research.

We investigated Callaway Carver, a nationally known therapeutic center for kids with developmental disorders. When we mentioned the place to Rhonda, she sniffed, "It's completely medicalized. They'll test and then put him on drugs. If that's what you want, I'll refer you. But they treat the kids like specimens."

Her opinion seemed biased, and, given her lack of results, we doubted it; but we didn't follow up because we still didn't grasp the severity of Cam's disorder. In fact, we told friends and relatives that he was "mildly autistic," and I was embarrassed even to use that phrase. The word "autism" seemed melodramatic, self-pitying, a word that would at first elicit sympathy, but soon earn boredom or contempt. I just knew Cam wasn't that impaired.

Yet other kids made his delays painfully obvious. One day at the playground, I encountered a neighbor whose precocious daughter was several months younger than Cameron. While my son aimlessly sifted sand, the little girl stood up, carefully smoothed her pink party frock, and announced, "My mom and dad eat cat food." Her mother shrieked with delight and mock embarrassment, then couldn't stop talking about how precious her daughter was.

From then on I avoided them, claiming that the mother was overbearing and self-centered. I didn't want to hear the truth. Then someone announced it so loudly that I had to pay attention.

In March 1993 we brought Cam to a highly reputed neurolinguist named Sarah Lincoln. A slender, cool woman in her late thirties, she watched our son "play," listened to our description of his problems, and tested his responses to various pictures. Cam mouthed objects and climbed on the furniture. As the evaluation proceeded, her manner became increasingly somber, and before long she looked as though she'd eaten something distasteful. At session's end, she briskly informed us that Cam had serious developmental problems and that we had a lot of work ahead of us. Then she tried to get rid of us as quickly as possible.

Her written report explains, "Cameron presents as a youngster with global sociolinguistic and communicative deficits, as well as many self-stimulating behaviors, consistent with a profile of autism/PDD." That was painful enough. But her final paragraph brought blood rushing to my face:

Clearly, Cameron is severely disordered in . . . his overall communicative and socio-linguistic drives and skills and not simply delayed. His inability . . . to participate in turn-taking behaviors makes formal assessment fairly useless and even observational developmental scales do not accurately depict this youngster's functioning. . . . Yet his occasionally purposeful eye contact and tolerance for attempts at interaction suggest he would benefit from intensive and directed teaching.

She recommended that Cam receive speech therapy and be placed in "a small, well-structured, highly language-focused preschool program" for developmentally delayed kids.

I tried to dismiss her assessment. "This is really harsh. I can't believe he's that bad. He identified the cup as 'coppee.' That's pretty good. I've never heard him say that before, have you? He also named 'ball.' Plus he was nervous and he doesn't do well under pressure. Geez, I don't think she saw anything good about him at all!"

Les said nothing. She looked sick.

I vehemently rejected Dr. Lincoln's report, but my denial was a thin veil over my real feelings: abject terror. I couldn't accept her evaluation. To do so would be to condemn us to a lightless horizon—no moon, no hope.

Not Otherwise Specified

But even if we had accepted Dr. Lincoln's recommendations, we had no idea how to follow them. What "small, well-structured highly language-focused preschool program?" Anyway, Rhonda insisted that Cam wasn't ready for a regular preschool. How could we get into such a program when Red Willow barred us?

This experience introduced us to problems that later became all too familiar: the politics of special education, the inadequacy of available resources, the absence of a central clearing house for information and referrals, and, most of all, the unreliability of "experts." We suspected that Rhonda didn't want to refer us elsewhere because she didn't want to lose a client. Did she like him especially well? Or couldn't she admit failure?

Soon we discovered Bernard Rimland's Autism Research Institute, and completed his diagnostic checklist for "Behavior-Disturbed Children." It asks some 200 questions to determine whether your child has autism. Some were designed to reinforce Rimland's pet theories about a relationship between autism and digestive problems. Others targeted classic symptoms: lining things up, waving fingers, fixation on objects, odd gait. Here at last, we felt, was a trustworthy instrument.

Two months later we eagerly scanned the results. A score of +20 or higher indicated classic autism, and children who score from -15 to +19, the report said, "are typically regarded as 'autistic' by professionals world-wide. The vast majority of children diagnosed as autistic fall within this range." Those who score -16 or lower are called "autistic-like" or some other nebulous description. Cam's scores? For behavior, -23; for speech -1, for a total of -24. Did this mean his prognosis was better? Or was it worse, since his differences from "classic" autism meant that nobody knew what to do with him?

I tried to feel encouraged: "See, he's not classically autistic!"

Les was more skeptical. "Look at the speech part, Wall. In terms of that, he's totally autistic."

Reviewing the sheet today reveals why such surveys have little value. We tried to answer honestly, but some responses reflect wishful thinking. For example, we claimed Cam was not excessively rigid—the boy who watched the same videos day after day. And we checked "no" to "covers ears at many sounds," even though he did so then and now.

That year we also treated Cam with Rimland's multivitamin and magnesium therapy. (The theory is that autistic kids can't metabolize certain vitamins, which worsens their cognitive and sensory problems. The magnesium is supposed to help them metabolize the vitamins and so reduce or eliminate some autistic symptoms.) For eight months we religiously sprinkled the foul-tasting powder into Cam's oatmeal or apple sauce. For weeks we said, "I think he *is* understanding more," or "Look, he seems calmer." But we were kidding ourselves. The therapy had no effect. The fact is, parents simply can't be objective about treatments: we see what we want to see. We wanted Cam to be less impaired, and denied what was obvious to others.

Around this time, a neighbor—the lady who had told us that Cam's "reading" was abnormal—recommended that we see Dr. Donald Archer. A lanky southerner in his sixties, he was Baltimore's most popular pediatrician, but he wasn't accepting new patients. I called his office anyway, explaining that Cam had autistic-like symptoms and that we hadn't been able to find a doctor to help us. To our surprise, Dr. Archer agreed to examine Cam. Later he explained why he'd made an exception. After serving in the military, he was older than most new medical students, so all of the schools to which he applied turned him down for being too old to handle the rigors of residency. But one school admitted him; its director had my last name.

Maybe things were turning our way!

We warned him that Cam might cause a scene, so he scheduled our appointment for after office hours. Dr. Archer listened to us recite Cam's problems, and performed other basic tests. He tried to get Cam to play with a ball and a toy, read a book to him, tested his speech.

For once an expert also talked to *us:* "I can see that you all have had a tough time. In the old days, they used to think that parents were to blame for autism. That was a tragedy. We know better now. In fact, most of the kiddos I've treated for this have very good parents who do everything to help their children. Just like you."

We asked if Cam's disorder could have been caused by his birth complications.

"Well, it's possible, but not probable. The research shows that a lot of the changes to these kids' brains occurs in areas that form early in prenatal development. Chances are that those parts were already programmed to go wrong by the time you had the placental abruption. Your body sensed that something was wrong; in a way it was trying to end the pregnancy." He turned his pale blue eyes sympathetically toward Les. "It's probably the opposite: the earlier developmental problems most likely brought on the birth complications."

We were oddly relieved—we hadn't done anything wrong.

I said, "He seemed normal when he was a toddler. In fact, he was precocious. He spoke his first word at ten months, and was 'reading' those toddler books at eighteen months old."

The doctor outlined a current theory that certain children's brains actually develop too fast. "It's like you're building a road through a wilderness. The fastest way to get from point to point is by a superhighway. But instead, for whatever biochemical reason, the brains of these kiddos go wild and build a whole bunch of little pathways. So it takes a lot longer for messages to get through. The accelerated growth, instead of helping them, actually messes things up."

His explanation was troubling: if Cam's neurology was already haywire, it might be impossible to fix it.

As we prepared to leave, Dr. Archer patted our son on the head and said, "You're an interesting fellow, Cameron." I thought grimly—as in the old Chinese adage, "May you live in interesting times." It's a curse.

He also handed us an invoice. Under "diagnosis" he'd written PDD-NOS. There it was again—"Pervasive developmental disorder, not otherwise specified." Something like autism, but not exactly. Was it better than autism? Worse? We seemed to have passed through the looking glass into a world where everyone spoke jabberwocky.

A physician had at last given us an honest and informed diagnosis. But it merely confirmed that the experts were as mystified by Cameron as we were. Our son had some disorder, but they couldn't or wouldn't name it. Meanwhile, the nameless thing was gaining power, defeating all attempts to drive it away.

Chapter 4

Raw Timber

Choose the timbers with greatest care;
Of all that is unsound beware
For only what is sound and strong
To this vessel shall belong.
—Henry Wadsworth Longfellow, "The Building of the Ship"

Special Needs

Les and I watch a speech therapy session from behind a one-way mirror. The therapist attempts to engage Cameron in a game of catch. But Cam doesn't catch on: he throws the ball back to the therapist once, then flings it at the wall and waves his fingers. Once he springs up to climb on the couch, glancing back at the therapist. "Loo, loo," he comments. "Hooka bookah." But most of time he just gazes at his hands or feet or the floor. If she moves the chair in which he is rocking or makes him stop climbing, he throws himself down, screams, and grabs her hair.

We had started twice-weekly speech therapy sessions at my college's clinic. A graduate student, supervised by a professional speech pathologist, outlined specific goals: increase Cam's turn-taking abilities, improve his eye contact, help him learn to use certain toys, enhance identification of objects. We were heartened.

But Cam's inability to pay attention, his utter lack of interest in games, his seeming incomprehension of the most elementary tasks, were excruciating to witness. As each session went sour, Les or I would enter the therapy room and offer tips ("first say, 'look at me, Cam,'" or "maybe we should start with something he likes"), but mostly we watched glumly from the other room. Our son's distractability and perseveration weren't deliberate, but it was hard not to *feel* that they were. Cam could sometimes complete these tasks at home, so why not here? He seemed so bright-eyed: why couldn't he express that intelligence?

Their final report sounded encouraging ("Cam is an energetic child who has enjoyed interaction with the clinician and progressed communicatively.... Cam has improved eye contact . . . and is beginning to develop turn-taking behaviors"), but we all knew his progress had been minimal.

In June 1993 we met with the Red Willow staff to create Cam's IEP. Among his listed "strengths" were: "comprehends 2-step directions, demonstrates verbal-communicative intent, can string beads, likes to jump, enjoys people he knows, matches objects, and recognizes familiar people." Calling these skills "strengths" in a four-year-old is stretching the word's meaning well beyond its typical range. But they had to say *something* positive.

In contrast, the "needs" column was packed with generalities. "To demonstrate an understanding of abstract concepts; to utilize meaningful intelligible verbal language; to integrate two hands in fine motor tasks." One could imagine how to address these goals. But what about "continue to develop age-appropriate skills," "learn to interact with peers," or "develop independent work skills?" The nebulousness of these goals pointed again to the severity of Cam's disability and his teachers' uncertainty about how to treat it.

The IEP team officially recommended "a small, highly structured special education program using a visually-based system of instruction such as TE-ACCH" (a task-completion pedagogy developed at the University of North Carolina). They also told us that, come fall, Baltimore County was starting a pilot program for kids with autism/PDD. We put Cam's name on the list and waited.

In the Mill

In August, Cam was accepted into the program. Timberland Elementary was the site for the only two classes in our section of the county. After learning he had been accepted, Les and I shared a congratulatory hug. At last our son would receive intensive teaching from knowledgeable people!

Before the term started, we met with the teacher, Donna DeMazio, and the program coordinator, Diane Corbett. Both seemed well prepared, and the

TEACCH program, which allows each child to move at his or her own pace, seemed well suited to Cam.

Still, we faced the first day of school with every parent's mix of trepidation and excitement. We were used to having him away from us at day care. But this was different: our boy was going to his first real school. We busied ourselves with preparations: book bag? Check. Supplies? Check. Face washed? Check. Teeth brushed? Check (sort of: he wouldn't hold still). My wife and I walked Cam to the bus, each firmly holding one of his hands, certain he'd bawl or throw a tantrum as it departed. Les gave him a pep talk: "Look at the big bus! It's going to take you to school! That will be so much fun!" But he didn't need it. As the bus departed, he placidly gazed out the window. Meanwhile, Mom and Dad were crying like little kids.

As months passed, Timberland began to remind me of the sawmill where I'd worked to earn money for college. Small children, all unformed aptitudes and unfocused energy, were processed like raw timber—graded, refined, graded again, then moved along the conveyor to the next stage. Each child was socialized and processed until his or her talents emerged. The few unsound or defective specimens—those for whom even special education isn't special enough—were culled and earmarked for the scrap yard. That, I feared, would be our son's future.

Cam couldn't regulate his attention; he was overstimulated; he couldn't grasp the daily sequence. The classroom was a barrage of blinding, skittering sensations and conflicting messages. Anxious, he lashed out; miserable, he made them share his misery.

His daily report included a column labeled "played with," and a check box beside each classmate's name. Only three times that year were any boxes checked. In his first quarter report, the teacher wrote, "In the toy area of the room he does not choose to play with toys with or near anyone else. If someone sits near him he will usually get upset."

His actual accomplishments were, to put it kindly, modest. For the first few weeks, the positive comments the teacher recorded in our take-home notebook were things like "sat for short times," "liked to climb," "made eye contact," and "less things in mouth." Under "free play," she wrote, "wandered and picked things off the floor" ("and put them into his mouth" was understood). One day, clearly puzzled, she wrote, "Does he play with anything at home?"

Occasionally a message would sweeten our day. In October, the teacher wrote that he answered "Moo," to "What does a cow say?" A few days later, he "spontaneously said 'banana' when he saw it."

The negatives? There were so many that she didn't bother to give details. Some days brought only a cryptic sentence: "Screamed more." One day in January: "Cam spent most of the day in the bean-bag chair. We had to put him in the corner for biting." The original goals template included a category for "decrease anxiety"; by the second month it had become grittier: "decrease hitting, hair-pulling, and biting." Other entries included "We worked intensely on not putting staples in mouth." As demands increased, so did his disruption. His academic progress? In March, the teacher recorded a score of 0/20 for expressively identifying pictures. How could Cam identify pictures when he wouldn't look at them? And why wouldn't he look at them?

Most of the objectives we'd established—"tell about a recent experience," "use feeling words," "verbally ask a peer to do something"—were far beyond Cam's reach. And the TEACCH model's focus on independence didn't fit; to make him concentrate for several minutes and then start over when he wasn't working independently was to ensure failure.

The speech pathologist's reports were no more encouraging. In early October, she wrote, "He imitates/repeats many words and I have even heard him repeat simple phrases. (If only I could understand everything he says!) He can answer some simple questions and responds to verbal directions (I have had to consistently use *no* when he attempts to bite). Cameron is not screaming as much to show anger—a good sign!" Whoopee!

Most positive reports were related to food, such as when he spontaneously said, "My cookie." One "positive" entry thrust a needle into my heart: "spontaneously said *crying*." What agony had forced *that* word from his mouth?

Near the end of the year, we completed a developmental checklist. In every category, we checked perhaps the first ten or fifteen, called a few "emerging," and crossed out the rest. Gross motor skills remained his strongest area: he could roll and catch a ball, pedal a tricycle, and perform other age-appropriate physical activities. Of the seventy items under "cognitive" (for example, "read shape words," "learn days of the week"), we checked twelve. That's 17 percent.

By the end of the year, Cam could sit still longer and do simple put-in tasks; his receptive language had improved from virtually zero to minimal. He made better eye contact. The teachers insisted that he'd had a good year.

The school photos for 1993–1994 tell a different story. Cameron was becoming a handsome boy, with light brown hair, big brown eyes, and, when he flashed it, an infectious smile. But in the yearbook photo, he looks anxious and glances suspiciously out the corner of his eyes. A Polaroid of him "playing" at school depicts the child we saw frequently—hands stiffly clapping, mouth pursed to say "ooohh"—a child in anguish.

Other Mothers

School introduced another new factor into our lives: other parents. We learned that parental competitiveness doesn't vanish when kids are disabled; it merely changes form. For one mother, it wasn't enough that her son Anthony, Cam's classmate, was developmentally delayed; she also insisted that her seemingly typical older son had Asperger's syndrome (then a new term for higher-functioning autism). She constantly complained about services Anthony wasn't getting, listed his problems, and revealed, in uncomfortable detail, their chaotic home life: "My husband, Martin, you know, he can't handle Anthony at all. He just closes off and goes to his room. And Gary picks on Anthony. Sometimes I have to slap his hands and say, 'Gary, leave Anthony alone. How would you like to be autistic?'"

She would loudly announce in public that her son was autistic and bought cards that read, "Please excuse me, I have autism." She'd phone Leslie in the evenings and launch into a long narrative about Anthony but lose interest when Les started talking about Cam.

At the time we found her extremely irritating, but she was simply scared to death. She needed validation; having a disabled kid gave it to her. If you can't beat autism, she seemed to have decided, why not turn it into a badge of honor? She may have had the right idea.

Cam did have one friend at Timberland—Jimmy Knowles, a sweet little guy with dark hair and enormous brown eyes whose passivity contrasted starkly with our own box of popping springs. Cam seemed to enjoy Jimmy's calm; the night before he returned to school from Christmas break that first year, Leslie heard him repeating, "Jimmy, Jimmy."

We visited his family several times and often compared notes over the phone. But it was difficult to air our views because Mrs. Knowles chattered compulsively.

"Did you guys get allergy testing?"

"Yes, we went through the first session on Monday."

"Oh, that's good, because we had Jimmy tested and of course he was allergic to everything. I told Tom that he's just like him, because Tom, you know, is severely allergic to trees. Oaks, I think. Anyway, all spring long he just sneezes and sneezes. I asked them if they'd put an air cleaner in the classroom, you know, to clean up all that dust floating around, and they just looked at me. I don't want to be pushy, but I think they should do everything they can to help these kids out. They don't need sneezing and runny eyes on top of everything else." She stopped for a breath.

"I know. We're trying just about . . ."

"Have you guys done that vitamin therapy? Someone said it really helped their kid—I think it was Angie Palmer, you know her? She has Aston, the big blond boy? You can just tell by looking that something's wrong with him! Anyway, we can't get Jimmy to eat much of anything except cereal and applesauce, so I crumble up the pills and give it to him with applesauce. I think it might be helping."

"We tried that, but it didn't work. In fact—"

"That's too bad. But Cam is so darling. Thank God they have that going for them. Sometimes Jimmy is so adorable and other times he just sits there like the village idiot."

During one conversation, Leslie implied that Jimmy and Cam might in fact be mentally handicapped. Mrs. Knowles vehemently denied it and never called us again.

Misbehaving

The next school year—1994–1995—brought an immediate uproar over Cam's aggression. Things were bad enough that in November we had to call a special "team" meeting.

Les was room mother that year, and after one classroom visit came home furious about the long stretches of unstructured time she had witnessed. When Cam finished his work bins, or during transitions, or whenever they couldn't get him to cooperate, they placed him in the "toy area," a 4' x 5' enclosure containing a few battered cars, blocks, and a few other toys. Nobody encouraged him to play, so essentially he was fenced in like a feral pup. We wrote back protesting Cam's being "penned up."

We offered other suggestions. Cam's visual perception was weak, so he didn't understand the picture symbols they used. We suggested they use an auditory schedule, or a Language Master (a machine that plays back phrases recorded on strips on a card). And wouldn't Polaroids work better than picture symbols to help Cam connect image and concept? Could they give him speech and occupational therapy during class time, rather than pulling him out for the sessions? We recommended music as a reward and tranquilizer. But the staff stubbornly clung to methods that weren't working and to a goal of independence that our son clearly could not meet.

One of the strangest phenomena was the staff's shoe fixation: note after note asked why Cam needed to remove his shoes. They seemed to believe that if he'd just keep his shoes on, why, all his problems would just disappear! Near the end of the year, without our knowledge, they began fastening them with duct tape (that practice ended as soon as we found out about it).

In that year's class photo, five neatly dressed boys sit in a row, and three actually face the camera. Next to the little sign—Timberland Elementary School, Mrs. DeMazio, 1994–1995—a pair of bare feet dangles in plain sight. They're attached to my son.

Shoes were only the beginning. By January, Cam was disrobing completely. Did the clothing textures bother him? Was it related to toilet training ("I have to take off my pants to pee, so I'll just keep them off all the time")? We speculated that this was Cam's solution to a sensory problem: though unsure about what he saw and heard, he trusted his sense of touch. Like a bug probing with antennae, he used his feet to gain information about his environment. Yet his teacher insisted on blocking his one dependable sense.

In fact, she often seemed obtuse. For example, we gave her one of Cam's favorite books, *Max's Christmas,* hoping it might help him remember how to read. The book is full of questions from the curious Max and answers from his officious big sister Ruby. Cam could gleefully supply the right answers if you prompted him with the questions.

After he's put to bed, Max sneaks down the stairs to wait for Santa. "Max waited a long time."

When I read the book to Cam, I always exaggerated the word so that Max has to wait a looooooooooooooooooooonnnnnnnnnnngggggggggggg. . . . Cam would giggle, squirm, and then add, "Tine." I'd make "long" even longer. "Tine!" he'd insist with a laughing shout.

A few months after Christmas the teacher returned the book. She'd replaced all the questions with a banal narrative: "Now the bunny puts the toys under the tree," and "Oh, look, the bunny fell asleep." Her "improvements" had destroyed Cam's interest and pleasure.

In the spring she wrote, "Does anyone in Cam's family speak French? He sings 'Frere Jacques' and says 'Louie, Louie' all the time. Today it sounded like he was trying to say something in French." But anybody who has worked with Cam for half an hour should know that "looie" is his happy sound. It simply means "I feel good." Was she even listening?

Ms. Corbett tried to stay positive. In November, she noted that she'd heard a good deal of spontaneous language: "go get in the car," "open the door please," "all gone." But she was grasping at straws: one day they played with bubbles, and the next she read him a story. In one entry, she wrote that they sang everything, yet in the next entry she had forgotten all about singing and was rewarding attention with snacks. No wonder Cam was confused. Her premolded patterns didn't fit his shape; he didn't belong in her mill.

That spring she complained about Cam's constant pinching; we responded with a memo outlining ways to handle it and implying that she may have prodded him too much. She dashed off an indignant note: "I think we are knowledgeable enough about Cam and his uniqueness *not* to be doing the things you suggest. . . . I am a professional in the area of processing . . . language, and understand the importance of 'wait time.' . . . All of which I don't need to be reminded of." We crafted a conciliatory reply, some of which we actually believed.

But we knew that Cam's worsening aggression wasn't all their fault. We believed it was related to a surge in cognitive development: he could think of more things but couldn't communicate them. Occasionally those thoughts came through. For example, in April Cam put his hand in the butter. Les said, "You need toast for butter." Cam answered, "We have toast." Another day Les asked, "Why are you biting?" Cam: "I like it." Most of the time, though, he seemed oblivious to words, which only made those glints of intelligence more frustrating.

Cam's school photo for that second year again reveals a great deal. He wants to please the adults but can't comprehend what he's supposed to do. Beneath his brave smile, he's about to burst into tears.

A year's worth of pain and frustration is etched on that little face.

Things Not Seen

Leslie began having a recurring dream. She's swimming with Cam when his head suddenly disappears. Panicked, she dives beneath the surface, but the dark, murky water conceals him. She gropes for an arm or leg, but Cam's limbs are out of reach. Her son is drowning and she can't save him. Then she wakes—into the same nightmare.

She did all she could. Our worst fear was that we'd look back in ten years and say, "Oh, I wish we'd tried *x*." If we just refused to surrender, just worked hard enough, we'd beat autism. So Les quit her job in October 1994 to devote herself to the battle. She became a dynamo. In addition to twice-weekly speech therapy and consultations with behavior specialists about Cam's aggression, she got him started on weekly sessions with a vision therapist.

Over several months, the therapist tried various measures—dropping balls from the ceiling, displaying a bank of lights and asking Cam to track them—but he invariably dashed for the bathroom (crying "potty," though he seldom needed to go) or darted into the waiting room to riffle through the eyeglass displays. Whenever a light came near him, he'd flop on his back and scream. During one session, he tried to slap the doctor. When Les intervened, Cam bit her arm.

The doctor maintained a good front, but her mask slipped one day as we chatted about bratty kids. Trying to reassure us, she confided, "I've seen kids who weren't handicapped behave just as badly. You see them one minute and they're sweet and the next they're like Cam or even worse. You know, Damien." She rolled her eyes, then blushed.

Cam's visual tracking improved a little, but this minimal progress had cost enormous effort, so after a few months we suspended the therapy. In her final report from May 1995, the doctor noted that Cam's aggression came from "trying to avoid or delay work which [he] knows is very stressful," and that "the behavior which looks like laziness or inattentiveness is actually a survival tactic." We'd known that much. But although she claimed he'd made "incredible strides" (for example, he could now place a peg in a hole and stack blocks), she was clearly just trying to make us all feel better.

A couple of parents had told us that their children's behavior had improved with allergy therapy, so we signed up for allergy testing with Dr. Timothy Payton. Maybe putting a stop to Cam's constantly runny nose and frequent earaches would help him focus.

We'd warned the nurses about Cam's inability to wait, so they gave us our own waiting room, into which we lugged Cam's Fisher-Price tape player and Raffi tapes, his books, and plenty of snacks. Every fifteen minutes, a nurse entered with a rack of tubes and needles, and pricked Cam on the arm and shoulder. A hive reaction to any of the pricks meant he was allergic, so they kept jabbing him with increasingly diluted solutions until he no longer displayed a hive. The tests went on for hours, and with every poke Cam screamed as though he were being knifed. When I later underwent allergy testing myself, I was surprised to discover that the needles didn't hurt. But to Cam they felt like bee stings.

Our son seemed to be allergic to everything, and the doctor put him on a regimen of two separate liquid formulas—one for molds and dust mites, and another for food allergies—to be taken twice a day under the tongue. We were certain we saw improvement in his allergies and general behavior, and his ear infections gradually abated.

A year later, I also took up Dr. Payton's regimen. After two years, however, I stopped and noticed no change at all. Later, we learned from a different allergist that a skin test couldn't reveal food allergies. In short, these tests (and probably the treatments) lacked scientific validity. We'd been afraid to stop giving Cam the drops because we wanted to believe we were helping him. But when we discontinued them Cam had no reaction. The treatments had cost over $200 a month: we'd thrown away more than $5,000.

Other tests were more revealing—and more frightening. In the spring of 1995, the school professionals administered Cam's post-kindergarten assessments. According to the teacher's evaluations, he was severely delayed in all areas except gross motor skills: "Cameron's overall developmental age on this assessment is 26 months." She measured Cam's IQ at 42.

The educational mill was either running backwards or not at all, the timber—our child—growing more raw. And he wouldn't stay green forever, because his brain would eventually lose its plasticity and harden into its current form.

I cast aspersions on her competence: how could the same teacher who'd had such a tough time with Cam for the last two years test him accurately?

But it wasn't as easy to dismiss the school psychologist's assessment. This man had noticed, during classroom visits, that whenever Cam threatened to bite or scratch, the teachers massaged or brushed him. He concluded that Cam manipulated them by faking aggression. He had recognized that our son wasn't too cognitively impaired to outfox some adults.

Yet he assessed Cam's developmental age at thirty-six months. Our son was then almost six, so that meant his IQ was around 50. Equally disturbing were the results of the CARS (Childhood Autism Rating Scale) he had administered. Cam had scored in the moderate to severe range.

"Moderate to severe?" I said indignantly, reviewing the report at our kitchen table. "No way. Mild to moderate, or maybe moderate, but severe? Impossible."

Les pointed out the astuteness of his other observations. "Moderate to severe," she said. "Oh, Bunny, those kids don't get better."

"Some of them do. Anyway, Cam is not severe. I just don't accept that. They have to lowball the kids so they don't give parents false hopes."

As I continued to rationalize and deny, Leslie just gazed at me, her brown eyes filling with tears.

Chapter 5

Golden Slumbers

Golden slumbers kiss your eyes
Smiles awake you when you rise
Sleep, pretty wantons, do not cry,
And I will sing a lullaby.
—Thomas Dekker, *Patient Grissil*

One evening while Leslie was pregnant with Cameron, I met three colleagues at a tavern to plan a course we were co-teaching. One of them, the father of a five-year-old daughter, advised me about what to expect once our child was born. Having heard horror stories about sleep deprivation, I casually asked, "What about sleep?"

A faraway look came into his eye as he pensively took a sip of his beer. "Ah, sleep. It's our most precious commodity." We all hooted, but he wasn't kidding. Even as a three- and four-year-old, his daughter couldn't fall asleep at night. They tried reading to her, telling her stories, playing music, rocking her; they tried keeping her up later and later; they threatened, cajoled, pleaded, and stormed. All to no avail. Finally her dad resorted to driving: the drone of the road eventually made his daughter drowsy.

So I was mildly apprehensive about this notorious phenomenon, but figured we could handle it. And we did. At first.

Wynken, Blynken, and Nod

By age three Cam had become an exhausting child. He wanted to climb on everything—kitchen table, living room chairs, and couch. When he wasn't climbing, he was jumping—on his trampoline, the couch, the bed. The rest of the time he stacked things, often dragging one chair to another and piling them up to provide a climbing perch. This constant exercise helped him sleep, so after 8 p.m. we generally enjoyed blessed respite from his relentless activity.

When we read about the "sleep problems" of many kids with autism, we smugly assumed that those parents must be doing something wrong.

Then suddenly everything changed: once he turned five, Cam couldn't buy a ticket to slumberland. We'd put him to bed with his usual comforts—music, his "B" (a tattered white baby blanket) and "suckie"—but soon he'd bound into the living room wearing a big grin: "Here I am!" We'd put him back to bed; he'd get up again. We'd put him back a little less gently; moments later we'd hear him bouncing on his bed or on his big gym ball.

"Cam, you need to get to sleep now, or you'll be tired in the morning. Then you won't have any fun, and you'll feel yucky. It's time to go to . . ."

"Sweep."

"That's right. Go to sleep. Ni-night."

"Night."

But he couldn't go night-night.

Night after night we played lullabies; night after night he watched his *Good Night, Sleep Tight* video; night after night we read him his favorite books. Night after night I'd recite "Wynken, Blynken, and Nod" with him, emphasizing its final lines:

> So close your eyes
> While Daddy sings
> Of wonderful sights that be
> And you shall see the beautiful things
> As you rock in the misty sea
> Where the old shoe rocks the fishermen three
> Wynken, Blyken, and Nod.

Winking and blinking were no problem; but Cam just could not nod.

At first patient, we soon grew irritated, and finally irate. On his third time arising each evening, Cam would tiptoe into the living room or sneak around the corner, trying not to alert us. When, at 10 p.m., he was still roaming his room or climbing on the furniture, we'd apply a gentle slap on the rump. "Damn it, Cameron. Now *go to sleep!*" Cam would bawl awhile, then drop off.

For several weeks in the summer of 1994, this little drama played out every night.

He seemed to need the release of a good cry before he could fall asleep. But that meant spanking him every night—not good. We were guilt-ridden, and Cam was getting increasingly anxious about bedtime. And so were we.

Then I read a *Newsweek* article about melatonin. Among its many virtues, the article claimed, was the capacity to induce sleep. A natural hormone produced by the pineal gland, it has no side effects. But where could you find it? I called pharmacies, health food stores, supermarkets. Most had never heard of it and none had it. (This was before a melatonin craze swept the country the following year.) Finally, I found a natural food store that stocked the supplement. A bottle of sixty tablets clutched in my hand, I raced home to share the good news.

But was it safe for kids? And what was the proper dose for a five-year-old? I consulted our medical guide; Les called our pediatrician. Nobody seemed to know, but all doubted it was harmful. And it certainly seemed preferable to spanking him every night.

That evening at 9 p.m., Les carefully cut one of the orange-flavored 3 mg pills in half and fed it to Cam. We cast worried glances at him every few seconds, checking for . . . something. Within twenty minutes, his lids were drooping; by 9:30 he was sound asleep.

It was a magic elixir!

Doubts still nagged: we desperately needed sleep, but couldn't shake the sense that dosing a small child with a pill every night violated the Good Parent Code. And we'd grown so accustomed to our nasty evening ritual that its absence now seemed strange. Nevertheless, for the next few months Cam took melatonin every night before bedtime, and by 9:45 he was with Wynken, Blynken, and Nod, rocking on the misty sea.

Dreaming of a Song

The next spring, Cam again stopped sleeping through the night. Sometimes he had urinated, but he was wearing pull-up pants, so something else was triggering his internal alarm clock at 1:45 or 3:30 or 4:09. After two or three restless nights, he'd conk out the next evening at 7:00 p.m. and sleep soundly until morning. But this early bedtime didn't solve the problem: early to bed meant early to rise. On such occasions, his morning, and ours, began at 5 a.m.

Was it the melatonin? The bedwetting? Was some sound waking him up? Bad dreams? Cam couldn't tell us.

We tried giving him the melatonin after 10 p.m., but then he'd wake up at 4:30, revved up and ready for the day. If we withheld the melatonin, he'd still be climbing and stacking at midnight. Our evenings became a reality-show version of *Night of the Living Dead,* our house a tiny castle besieged by a one-child army. Sometimes Les and I just left him in the living room and sullenly retired. Whoever pretended most stubbornly to be asleep wouldn't have to get up with Cam. After a couple of nights, the one who'd been getting up would testily shake the other, "Hey, your turn!"

We had different methods of coaxing Cam into slumberland. My approach was to put him back to bed, play a classical music or lullaby tape, and lie beside him, talking softly.

"Cam, let's just relax," I'd whisper. "Listen to that music. It's so nice." I'd stroke his back and hold him tightly. Once his breathing slowed, I'd carefully climb out and tiptoe back to our room. Occasionally it worked. But more often, as soon as I sneaked out of bed, Cam would giggle and dash into the living room.

Les's approach was to give him something to eat or put on a video. Her tactics also worked occasionally but no more often than mine. Sometimes we switched. Either way, Cam's insomnia continued.

We tried obstinately remaining in bed to force him to entertain himself or fall asleep on his own. But Cam would clap loudly, pound on the walls, splash in the toilet, or urinate on the rug or couch. Translation: "Wake up, Mom and Dad!"

My friend's words no longer seemed funny. Now Les and I made our own grim jokes: "You want to soften up a suspect? Three nights with Cam and you'll confess to anything."

The cycle became self-perpetuating. When you're awakened for several nights running, your sleep rhythms are thrown out of whack. So even on the rare nights when Cam did stay asleep, I was plagued with insomnia, unable to turn off my internal sentinel. *When will he wake up? What'll I do when he does?*

Back when I played music full-time, I used to key myself down after gigs by making up set lists and mentally playing through them. Now, however, I got stuck on a single tune, often ones I didn't even like (for example, Bob Seger's "Night Moves") or that seemed to mock my plight, like The Beatles' "I'm Only Sleeping" ("Lying there and staring at the ceiling / Waiting for a sleepy feeling"). For one whole week, I fixed on the old standard "Stardust," my mind a CD player set on endless repeat: "Sometimes I wonder why I spend the lonely night / Dreaming of a song." After hours of musical torture, I'd open one eye and peer blearily at the clock: 2:48.

Thus did I grow intimately familiar with the insomniac's paradox: the inability to sleep is caused by the fear of not getting to sleep. The more you think about sleep, the less you can do it. The problem seemed to symbolize our life with autism: one vicious cycle after another.

We realize now that we should have alternated evenings on duty, or set up a cot in the basement so one of us could sleep away from the noise. Maybe our minds were fuzzy from lack of sleep, but more likely we just couldn't believe the pattern would continue. To accept that Cam's sleep problems might endure would be to admit that he was really autistic.

I wasn't ready to concede this truth.

In June 1995, following Cam's second year in Mrs. DeMazio's class, I was scheduled to give a paper at a conference in Providence, Rhode Island. We decided to make it a family vacation and drive up the coast from Baltimore. This trip was the catalyst that broke the cycle.

All three of us stayed in a single hotel room, which meant that every evening Cam stayed awake until at least 11 p.m. He couldn't put together a puzzle, use a crayon, play board games, or even watch TV for more than five minutes, unless it was one of his videos. Instead he bounced on the bed, pulled the blankets off, ran water, splashed it everywhere, then gulped mouthfuls (which made him pee), took extra baths, pounded on the windows and walls, and yanked on the draperies.

Sometimes Les took him for a run down the hotel corridors. During one of these excursions, Cam spotted an open door and, yelping with pleasure, scampered into the inviting room. Wide-eyed, Les followed him through the door.

A thirtyish couple and their two small children were lined up against the wall like hostages at a bank robbery, staring in disbelief at the five-year-old giddily bouncing on their bed.

Les handled it with aplomb. "Hi, I'm Leslie and this is my son Cameron. He's autistic, so he doesn't have any common sense. I was letting him run the halls for exercise. I'm sorry if he disturbed you. . . ."

"That's okay," the man said, smiling sheepishly.

"Okay, Cam, let's go!" But Cam wasn't about to give up that easily; he bounced higher and higher, his grin growing wider with each bounce. Finally, Les set her jaw, snatched him in mid-bounce, and tucked him under her arm like a halfback carrying a football. Cam writhed and howled in protest as she made her way to the door—"Sorry to intrude. He doesn't mean any harm. Well, bye!"—and scuttled back to the room where I'd been enjoying a shower, oblivious to their adventure.

Amazingly, Cam could sleep in a hotel room. We'd read until he fell asleep and then retire around midnight. We'd all wake up around 7:30. When we returned home, I no longer had insomnia and Cam slept through the nights.

He still couldn't get to sleep until after 10 p.m., but we were willing to sacrifice our R and R for some REM. Gradually we worked the melatonin back in, so that by the time school started that fall, we'd reached equilibrium. We cautiously began to relax.

The Potty Train

That fall we took him out of diaper pants, and when he awakened in the morning, he'd walk to the bathroom and urinate—all with only minimal prompting. But in March 1996, for no apparent reason, he started wetting the bed. We kept hoping this new behavior would just go away. No such luck.

A typical night went like this.

It's 3:34 and I hear clapping. "He peed the bed again. Shit!" I throw the covers aside and stumble into Cam's room. He stands there, pretending to ignore the drenched blankets and yellowish puddle on the mattress cover. He looks up fearfully at the red-eyed ogre who has barged into his room. I clap a paw on his shoulder. "Do you need to go potty?"

"Potty."

"Then get your butt in there!"

I hustle him into the bathroom. We wait five minutes, as he dutifully stands on the cold tile floor, trying to void an already empty bladder. He gazes up at me for approval or comfort. I can't give it to him. Hands trembling, he stares back at the toilet. At length I hear a fine stream of urine trickle timidly into the bowl.

"Is that all?"

"Ah."

I squat next to him. "Look at me."

His wandering eyes briefly rest on mine. "When you have to go potty, get out of bed!"

As soon as I say these words, I realize how absurd they sound: he *is* getting out of bed. He probably doesn't even understand what he's done wrong; all he knows is that Dad is very mad.

Back in his bedroom, I yank off Cam's wet blankets and cover him with clean ones. "Now get back in bed and go to sleep." I tuck him roughly between the covers and pull the door closed with a not-quite slam.

And that's a good night.

He lies awake, petrified he'll wet the bed again, frightened of his angry father. A half-hour later he walks into the bathroom and pees on the floor, or pads into the living room and piddles on the rug. Then he dashes around the living room clapping his hands, turning on lights, slapping the walls. Leslie and I wait each other out. Eventually one of us arises and puts Cam back to bed. Not gently. Cam is no longer toilet trained, but Les and I are fully trained to get up almost every night.

Some nights, Les and I just lie there as he yells, throws himself back on the bed, flips the lights on and off, drums on the windows, runs water in the sink or bathtub. The hell with it. We can't move. All we can think of is getting some shut-eye.

We know now that we should have ignored the bedwetting. Instead of scolding our son, we should simply have changed his bedclothes and put him back

to bed. But when you're in the center of a typhoon, you don't stop and take lon-
gitudinal bearings. So we foolishly clung to misguided ideas about discipline
that were making our lives miserable.

Strangely, the lack of sleep didn't seem to affect Cameron. Unlike his chronically tired, short-tempered, and groggy parents, Cam behaved no worse when
he'd been up most of the night than when he'd enjoyed a full night's sleep. If
anything, the days when he was tired were better than others: sleep deprivation
slowed his perpetually revving internal engine. He was calmer at school and
more compliant at home. But manageability was poor compensation for our
bedraggled days and edgy nights.

After months of this struggle, we altered our routine. Now when Cam got
up, one of us would doze on the living room couch while he watched videos.
At 5 a.m. we'd put the sleepy boy back to bed and try to catch the night's final,
fleeting Z's. Some mornings found Mommy or Daddy and Cam asleep on different sections of the couch.

Still, Cam's sleep problems had become our marital problem. Evenings I'd
cloister myself in the den or disappear downstairs. Leslie, who had returned to
work in the fall of 1995, spent more and more time there, dreading the wild
child and resentful husband waiting at home. Recriminations were constant
companions, fellow passengers on the autism train.

If my sleep habits were intermittently derailed, Leslie's were completely
wrecked. Upon arriving home she'd slump, exhausted and rheumy-eyed, on
the couch, trying to stay awake. But the demands of her high-pressure job, too
many sleepless nights, and Cam's relentless needs often overcame her good intentions. I'd say nothing, knowing my silence would jab a guilt needle into her
but unable to care.

One evening, as Les lay on the sofa with her eyes closed, I saw what the ordeal
had done to her. Her olive skin had become drawn and waxen, her mouth fixed
in a frown. Where was the vivacious, confident woman who, two years after we'd
moved to Atlanta, had walked into the *Atlanta Journal-Constitution* offices and,
with no credentials other than guts and intelligence, landed a job that very day?

In June 1996 we had a talk.

"I can't live like this," she said. The circles under her brown eyes bore witness.

"I know it." I shrugged. "But we've tried everything. I swear it's related to the
bedwetting."

"Well, hollering at him when he wakes up isn't helping. He can't help it. God!
I don't know who's more stubborn, you or him."

She made a proposal: "Let's put him back in pull-up pants."

"No way. That would be giving up on toilet training. Anyway, he pees through
the pants."

"I don't care. I have to start getting some sleep. I'm sick all the time, I'm bone-tired, and my performance at work is awful. I'm drinking caffeine all day and guzzling wine at night to come down. I'm becoming Elvis, for Christ's sake!"

I gave a half smile. Yes, we were both all shook up. A long pause ensued while we stared at the walls. If we put him back in diapers, we'd lose the toilet battle; if we didn't, we might never again enjoy a full night's sleep.

"I just don't get it," I said. "We went through the entire fall and he didn't wet the bed once. Why did it change?"

"You know the answer: he's autistic."

There was nothing more to say. That evening we found the diaper pants we'd stored in his closet and put a pair on Cam. It worked. The pull-ups soaked up enough urine so he didn't wake up when he peed in them. We had our sleep back.

Our Most Precious Commodity

Cam's sleep problems never entirely disappeared. For the next several years, we usually put him to bed by 9:30, but he rarely dropped off until 10:30 or later. So what? Well, for one thing, we had to give up our evenings. Why couldn't we go into another room, read, or watch TV? Because Cam would pee on the floor or couch or break something. Instead we killed time, flipped through magazines or stared for the thousandth time at Raffi or *Mary Poppins*—waiting for one more endless evening to pass.

But at least we slept.

Cam's second bout of insomnia was related to toilet-training anxiety. But what about the other times? Did the wind blowing through the trees sound like a hurricane? Was he startled when a neighbor closed a car door? Did he have a bad dream?

I often wondered what dreams come to a child who understands so little language and even less about human behavior. Do his dream people speak in gibberish, like Alice's Wonderland friends? Does he replay his daytime rituals? Does he fantasize about being able to talk fluently, think clearly, and behave as others do? Does he even know they're dreams? Perhaps not: occasionally Cam leaps from his bed, enraged and ready to attack, seemingly shocked by a bad dream he believes is real.

Cam's waking life has often been a nightmare. No wonder he can't always distinguish dreams from reality. But in later years his nights have been mostly peaceful. Sometimes, after he's finally dropped off, I tiptoe into his darkened room and listen to the even breaths he draws through slightly open lips. Standing by his bed, I imagine my son's thoughts, ruefully recalling how we couldn't feel his suffering through the haze of our fatigue and frustrated hopes.

As I watch him sleep so serenely, I understand again how he has transformed our world into a mirror of his own: a solitary land, only occasionally brightened by peace and joy. Thus does an autistic child transfigure a family, remaking it in his own image.

Gazing down again at the slumbering figure, I sing, in a hoarse whisper, "Sleep, pretty darling, do not cry." Then I kiss his head and quietly close the door.

Chapter 6

The Thing with Feathers

Hope is the thing with feathers
That perches in the soul,
And sings the tune without the words,
And never stops at all . . .
—Emily Dickinson

Counting Down

One day in the fall of 1994, I returned from the library, dropped my briefcase with a crash and shouted for Les; I could barely contain my excitement. I had brought home a book by O. Ivar Lovaas, called *The Autistic Child: Language Development through Behavior Modification,* which documents his method of behavior modification/discrete trial teaching. Lovaas's results were phenomenal: many of his autistic patients actually recovered! We had to get this for Cam—the sooner the better.

Through the local Autism Society of America chapter, we obtained the name of a woman whose daughter was doing Lovaas therapy. The woman raved about it and referred us to the Blair School in New Jersey, which would send a supervisor to your home to set up a program and train parents and therapists. We completed the enrollment forms and put Cam's name on the lengthy waiting list.

The Timberland folks discouraged us: "their techniques are too mechanical," "kids can't be drilled that much," "the kids don't generalize." We ignored them; we no longer trusted their judgment.

When, several months later, the Blair School called to set a date for our initial workshop, our high spirits weren't deflated even by the stiff fee. Leslie had quit her job that fall, and without her income, we'd be hard-pressed to meet the expenses. So we took a leap of faith: we'd been contributing to a mutual fund earmarked as Cam's college savings. But it was already obvious that Cam wouldn't be going to college unless a miracle occurred, and this money might bring about that miracle. We withdrew the cash to use it for the Lovaas program.

For our initial workshop in February 1995, we recruited three therapists, all of them grad students in speech pathology. Our supervisor was Diane Ellison, a stocky, somewhat intimidating ex-Navy noncom who had retained her military bearing.

She briskly introduced us to Lovaas principles: begin with "come here" and "look at me," work incrementally from the most basic tasks and gradually teach the child to generalize and increase his attention span. Be friendly but firm and avoid inadvertently reinforcing unwanted behaviors. Give prompt reinforcers—food, praise, high fives—and vary them so the effects don't fade. Respond with a firm "no" for aggression and noncompliance. Take accurate and complete data.

Lovaas therapy (more generally called Applied Behavioral Analysis, or ABA) uses operant conditioning in discrete trials: the child repeats one drill and receives a reinforcer until he or she successfully completes a set number of trials, then moves to the next drill. You return to each drill at every session, but change the order so the child doesn't get locked into habits or memorize the order and begin to resist drills he hates. The method helps autistic kids understand when they've succeeded and allows plenty of breaks to accommodate their erratic attention spans. Above all, it provides clear and immediate rewards for successful work.

Diane spoke rapidly while we furiously took notes. After outlining the first drill, she squatted in front of Cam: "Cameron. Look at me." He waved his long fingers near his right eye and giggled.

"No," she said sharply, pulling his chin directly in front of hers. "Look at me."

He made fleeting eye contact.

"Good!" The drill sergeant became a rough-and-tumble big sister. She tickled his ribs. He gazed at her, mouth slightly open: is this a game? Is she going to hurt me?

She repeated the drill. This time he made eye contact right away.

"Great job, Cameron!" Diane enthused. "Give me five!" Cam tentatively raised his hand and Diane slapped it.

And so it began.

At first we were overwhelmed. There was so much to remember! But Diane's final words drowned out any misgivings: "Right now he's behind the other kids. But we're going to work hard and by the time he's seven, he'll be caught up."

Caught up!

Still, our novice therapists seemed dazzled, so Les gave them a pep talk.

"There's a lot to learn, but everything is all written down. We'll follow the plan and meet once a week to review and keep everybody together."

Faced with their uncertain smiles, she broke into an old high school cheer: "You can do it," clap, clap, clap, "yes you can!" clap, clap, clap.

Everyone laughed, but by the end of that first day we did think of ourselves as a team. We were going to beat Cam's autism. We could do it! Yes we could!

Taking Wing

Leslie organized the program with her typical skill and zeal. She created a schedule, compiled the list of programs, wrote sheets with the "SDs" (that is, directives, such as "put with same" or "do this"), bought toys, puzzles, cups, and games. She set up a data workbook and bought each therapist a white smock on which she had stenciled "Cam's Crew." We emptied the spare room where she'd kept her office and reserved it for Cam's sessions.

Ideally, you're supposed to provide thirty to forty hours of therapy per week. But with Cam already in school half-days, we didn't have that many hours available and couldn't afford them anyway. So we started with a two-hour session each weekday, plus three or four sessions each weekend, for a total of twenty hours each week. That was our financial limit and, we felt, the limit of Cam's endurance.

Once we'd succeed in getting Cam to come to the table on command—a two-week struggle—the next challenge was inducing him to look at the therapist. The problems that had plagued our home sessions two years earlier immediately reappeared. His attention was completely scattered: told to assemble a puzzle, he'd wave his fingers, clap and vocalize, pull the therapist's hair. He couldn't imitate an action without a physical prompt, and he resisted prompts.

Nevertheless, he made immediate gains. At the beginning, he couldn't put a single puzzle piece in its proper place; within a month he could put together a three-piece puzzle in seconds. Within three months, he was completing fifteen drills per two-hour session, including color/shape and letter matching, nonidentical sorting, "touch same" (hold up a blue square, place another on the table, and choose the proper color), ball play, a picture-matching game, nonverbal and verbal imitation. By summer, Cam was matching everything in sight.

Building on these skills, however, was a different story. Though he could imitate two-word phrases (Therapist: "red ball." Cam: "ball"; "Listen: *red* ball." "Reball"), if you held up a ball and asked him "What is it?" he couldn't consistently name it without a prompt. He'd stare at you as if hoping to read the word on your face. Then he'd start guessing. Usually the first answer was "orange," probably because the first item he'd successfully identified was an orange.

Any drill demanding sophisticated language skills befuddled him. Frustration made him hate the drill, which led to noncompliance; forcing him to come to the table prompted aggression, which made him dread the drill even more. Another vicious circle.

Yet, for the first time in his life our son was learning academic skills and remembering some of what he'd learned. Our fledgling was taking wing, and as he started to fly, hope emerged from its cave and commenced singing.

Our therapists were learning as much as Cam was. Playful but demanding Sharon was the leader, but Penny was nearly as good. Both were tough, and they needed to be: at five and a half, Cam already possessed a vise-like grip and didn't hesitate to pinch an arm or pull a fistful of hair when frustrated. Neither woman was fazed by his aggression.

We soon became Lovaas true believers and altered our speech clinic sessions to mirror the home sessions. We videotaped one session in April 1995.

An attractive child with long eyelashes and glossy, light brown hair, Cam wears an orange T-shirt and jeans. He works barefoot.

Even the preliminaries are designed to encourage speech. When he requests cheese, Sharon gives him an unopened package of string cheese. He hands it back to her. "What do you want me to do?" she asks.

"Open 'a cheese," he answers. She opens it and hands it to him; he devours the cheese.

He reaches for a cup and realizes it's empty.

"Cup o' water."

"Do you want a cup of water?"

"Uh yeah, uh yeah."

"Say, 'open the water.'"

"Open water."

"Help me pour."

"Pwaasshh," he whispers in a growl.

She faces him knee to knee for nonverbal imitation. "Do this." She claps. Cam laughs and claps.

"Do this." She touches her hair. Cam stares, giggles. "Do this." She stomps her feet. He makes a minimal foot movement.

"Yeah, I saw that!" She tickles him. The drill continues, but Cam is more interested in making spit.

"Ah done!" he says, looking hopefully up at Sharon.

"No, we're not all done. Got to keep working," she says brightly.

Cam grabs her knees and says, "Huh-uh huh-uh huh-uh." Then he looks directly into her eyes and announces, "Potty."

"You don't need to go potty; you just went, you silly," she says, tickling him under the arms.

He imitates clapping once more, then gets to "go play," which for him means roaming the room and checking out the empty water cup.

Next comes sorting: he's supposed to place laminated shapes into different bowls. Things go well for about five trials, and then he reaches back to yank on Sharon's shirt.

"No. Sort," she says neutrally. He throws his head back to butt her and bites the bowl. Sorting continues anyway, though he occasionally gnaws the cards or grabs at Sharon. Once he's finished, she tickles him.

He gets up to retrieve a plastic see-saw.

Sharon asks, "Want the up-and-down? What do you want to do?"

"Up and down," he chants. Sharon pushes him back and forth for a couple of minutes. He grabs her shirt again.

"No," she says firmly.

Next is color matching. But Cam wants music. "Piyer," he sings; that is, "Eensy Weensy Spider," the song cued on his tape player. Sharon keeps him on task. "Twinkow, twinkow," he sings: "Twinkle, Twinkle, Little Star" follows "Spider" on his tape.

"Put with same," says Sharon. Cam whimpers, bites the colored square, scratches her hand.

"No. Put with same." More matching, biting, scratching. Sharon persists and Cam eventually places all squares where they belong.

He looks for the tape player. "Twinkoh, twinkoh."

"Bring me the music," Sharon says. Cam walks over and picks up the ball. "No, music. It's over here." He can't find it, so she takes it and places it on the table. "Come over here and listen."

Cam begins wildly slapping her hair and shoulders. "Huh-uh, huh-uh, huh-uh, huh-uh!"

"Hands down," she commands. Cam latches onto her hair and tries to bite her head.

"Ah, I let you get me," she says, trying to sound unperturbed, though her flushed cheeks betray the effort behind her self-control. She detaches his hands and helps him play the tape. A couple of minutes pass.

"Time to work" is followed by more grabbing and pleading for "Piyer." After they finish two more drills, they play the song, and Sharon helps Cam imitate the spider's path.

Next is block-stacking, but by this time—they've been working for twenty-two minutes—Cam is wailing in earnest. Using light tickles as the reward, Sharon coaxes him to complete the drill.

"Take your shoes off," Cam announces. He means "put your shoes on," which signals the end of the session. Smiling hopefully, he walks to the door and holds the knob.

"Come here," says Sharon. He whines and grabs her shirt.

Next, Cam is asked to follow verbal commands by touching parts of the room. "Go to the door," says Sharon. He touches it, growling all the while. More tickling ensues. He chews his shirt, slaps at Sharon's knee. "Go to the door," she repeats.

Cam screeches.

"Go to the door."

He turns off the lights. Clever boy: if they can't see, they'll have to stop.

"Take your shoes off," he insists.

After the last drill—ball play, during which Cam bites the ball before each throw, as if punishing it for inflicting this torture upon him—Sharon finally utters the longed-for phrase: "All done, Cam," she says and waves.

"Bye-bye," Cam answers, scampering out the door.

This session was below average, with more disruption and aggression than in most home sessions. Even so, Cam completes every drill with some success. He speaks several intelligible three- and four-word phrases, and clearly indicates what he wants.

There was no doubt in our minds: we were on our way.

Cam's Crew

Autism is called a spectrum disorder, which means that affected people display a broad range of abilities. The Lovaas program introduced us to another spectrum—the wide array of personalities found in therapists, who were invariably female. Though this was a self-selected group—most had chosen "helping" professions such as speech pathology or special ed, so were altruistically inclined—the disparities were striking. There were soft-hearted junior moms who didn't follow the program but inspired Cam through love; there were fun-loving gals who approached sessions as games; there were grim girls who acted as though they were getting a bad grade if Cam couldn't complete a drill. Cam brought out the best in some and the worst in others; he was a mirror reflecting each one's needs and flaws.

The best were like patient, firm, vivacious Sharon. She was dedicated beyond all expectations. In January 1996, for example, a blizzard dumped two feet of snow on a city unaccustomed to winter weather. Traffic was paralyzed; our street wasn't plowed for several days. But though the roads were impassable, at 12:10 the day after the storm we heard a knock at the door; there was Sharon, bundled in an enormous parka, her nose and cheeks red from walking the half-mile through the snow drifts from her apartment to our house.

"Sorry I'm late," she said. As we gaped in astonishment, she shrugged. "I wasn't doing anything anyway, and I figured you guys could use a break." Whatever we paid her wasn't enough.

But other therapists took Cam's aggression or noncompliance personally and would scold him or start to cry. Others dutifully completed all drills but never smiled, thus ensuring that Cam felt oppressed. Still others fudged by not bothering with the most difficult drills. As the months passed, our expectations grew more modest; as long as a therapist showed up regularly, we didn't say much.

After Les went back to work in the fall of 1995, the daily duties fell mostly to me. My first big test came in the summer of 1996. A typical day went like this: 10 to 12: work session. Eat lunch, then go outside and swing or watch a video. Sessions from 1 to 3 p.m. and 3:30 to 5.

Why didn't I just teach Cam myself? Because I wanted so badly for him to succeed that I gave him severe performance anxiety. Nor could I always conceal my frustration when he didn't successfully complete a drill that I knew he could do. In any case, we eventually figured out that one of the benefits of Lovaas therapy is giving respite to stressed-out parents.

While the sessions went on upstairs, I usually worked in my basement office; but it was hard to concentrate on research while keeping an ear cocked upstairs for warning sounds. At least twice a week, I'd hear shuffling or squeals, then dash upstairs to detach Cam's fingers from a therapist's hair or shirt. I'd assess the situation. Is he hungry? Just delaying? Does he need a break? Often I could bring him back to earth with a rapid-fire nonverbal imitation drill that forced him to look and listen closely to me.

I often fretted that a mellower father, a father less focused on his career or less determined that his child succeed, would have halted the sessions when they hit rough patches. That father would have sacrificed his job for his kid. But work was my refuge. Without it, autism would have consumed my entire life instead of just most of it. Reading, writing, and preparing for classes let me carve out a small space where order and sanity prevailed.

We brought to the program our faith in the redemptive power of work. The Lovaas literature was full of stories about how parental persistence had paid off, so we weren't going to be defeated by anything so trivial as exhaustion or scratches. Any day might bring the big breakthrough! Besides, keeping Cam hard at work chased away some of the guilt that followed us everywhere like a hungry dog.

Finding and keeping therapists was nonetheless a chronic problem. When interviewing prospects, we were candid about Cam's aggression, but nothing could really prepare them for the onslaught. In 1996 and 1997, we placed ads in local college psychology and speech pathology departments. They featured a photo of Cam in a blue overcoat, smiling pleasantly while standing at our back door. The caption read, "I Have Autism and I Need Your Help." It was artfully designed to tug at youthful heartstrings. But word of mouth must have spread the news that our child was difficult, for this ad netted zero therapists.

Just as we had to learn to decode what Cam was trying to say through aggression or noncompliance, we also had to interpret therapists' nonverbal messages. Bruises, scratch marks, disheveled hair—these signs were easy to read. Others were more cryptic.

A strange form of blackmail evolved between us and the therapists. We felt guilty for subjecting these young women to our aggressive child. And they knew we'd have a tough time replacing them, so they had us at their mercy: we needed them more than they needed us. We often had to swallow our anger and indignation when they took advantage of this fact.

Few of the therapists possessed Sharon's dedication; not many treated it as a real job. Some were chronically late. Countless times I'd expect a therapist at 4 p.m. so I could attend a meeting or a rehearsal; but 4:15, then 4:30 would pass while I fumed, muttered, and paced, frustrated as much by my helplessness as by the therapist's tardiness. My anxiety would rub off on Cam, who'd be irritable by the time the therapist showed up.

Others took days off on short notice: "This is the weekend we always go to the beach," or "Since it's spring break, I'm going to stay in New Jersey for the next two weeks."

"Oh. Well, we really need you those days, but if you can't make it, I guess we'll stumble through." We dared not reveal our neediness for fear of scaring them off for good.

I had to remind myself constantly that they were, after all, just kids, and we were lucky they were, for no adult would subject herself to such punishment for the measly six, then eight, and then ten bucks per hour we could afford to pay. They weren't in it for the money but for the experience and because, God bless them, they loved Cam and wanted to help him.

And so the blackmail worked both ways. We were desperate people, and these soft-hearted women often yielded to our pleas for more work even when they didn't want to. For instance, Andrea, one of our most patient and intelligent therapists, left us to attend grad school. A few months later she called to see how Cam was doing; we invited her over, and within an hour had rehired her. Eventually she simply stopped showing up: it was the only way she could tear herself away.

Despite the problems, Cam brought out the best in most therapists. The superwomen, the little moms, the fun gals, the tough chicks, even the merely competent and reliable: they all deserve medals.

Crimes and Misdemeanors

The good therapists far outnumbered the bad. But inevitably, a few crew members were incompetent or untrustworthy. Laura, a slightly older woman who had worked with Cam at school, one day took Cam for a drive after a session. They returned almost an hour late.

"Boy, am I glad you're back," I said to her. "I was getting worried. Is everything okay?"

"Cam's fine, and I'm okay." I noted her messy hair and smeared mascara.

"Oh-oh. What happened?"

"We had a little problem. A . . . well, a car accident, a minor one. As we were driving back Cam started to get really worked up. He was kicking the seat and then he grabbed my hair." She sniffed; tears welled in her gray eyes. "I was trying to calm him down, but I ran a red light and then we hit somebody."

"What? You ran into a pedestrian!" My heart began to pitch.

"No, I mean we ran into another car."

"Jesus, you mean Cam caused a wreck!"

"Well, kind of. I should've been watching the road better. But he was getting real upset and kicking the seat, and I was trying to keep him from grabbing my hair!" Her voice trembled.

I opened the car door to let my son out. He testily said, "Aauuooh," but seemed okay.

As Laura filled in the details, I realized that a more resourceful person would have pulled over, bought Cam a drink, and waited until he calmed down before driving. But I couldn't blame her: we'd asked her to do too much before she was ready and were damn lucky they hadn't been seriously hurt—or worse. She had smashed up her car's right fender. We paid the $500 deductible for her body work. If only our psyches had been as easily mended.

Our doubts increased as most of her sessions went sour. One day I returned home to discover that Cam had removed all the light bulbs over the bathroom sink. Where had she been during this experiment? Against our better judgment we kept her; we had therapy slots to fill.

Then one day she wrote in the notebook: "I don't feel very comfortable working at home with Cam after the last few weeks (first when he hit me with the paddle, then getting head-butted on Mon).”

Cam had exposed her true nature; he had, in effect, fired her.

But even with her flaws, Laura couldn't hold a candle to Sheila McBride, who entered our lives in the spring of 1996, when we hired her to replace Cam's school aide. A wiry, birdlike woman in her forties, Sheila was an ex-nun whose resume listed years of experience in teaching. She even had disabled siblings.

She worked out well at school, so we soon employed her as a reserve Lovaas therapist. After her second day on the job, she asked to take Cam for a drive. All of our other therapists had sometimes done that, so I didn't anticipate a problem. But when, two hours later, they were still gone, I became quietly frantic. What did I really know about this woman?

A few minutes later, Sheila and Cam drove up in her battered gray Mazda.

“Geez, where were you guys?” I asked, trying not to sound angry.

Sheila bit her nails and patted Cam's head. “Oh, I took him to Discovery Zone.”

Cam got overstimulated even at Chuck E. Cheese's, where he once got stuck in a tunnel and refused to come out until Les crawled inside to extract him. It was far too early in our relationship for her to take such risks. I frowned.

“He certainly has lots of energy,” she continued, her voice betraying no sign of guilt, though she wouldn't look at me. Was her blankness a pose, or was she really so oblivious to boundaries?

“You were there the whole time?”

“No. I took him to the playground, and over to where I live, and then over to the school.” She flashed a brittle smile and snapped her head up and down, her eyes fixed somewhere behind my right shoulder.

This incident sowed doubts about Sheila's judgment. The doubts blossomed when she started showing up unannounced in the evenings carrying shopping bags full of games, finger paints, crayons, and exercise books she had purchased. She would enter the house—usually at dinner time—and plop these things down on the kitchen table, her face darting from mine to Leslie's as if searching for approval.

We were nonplused. “Wow, Sheila, thanks. This is all valuable stuff. How much was all this?”

“Oh, you don't have to pay me. Really, I'm glad to help out.”

After bestowing her gifts, she'd chatter on, offer to work more hours, and ask to come by in the evenings and take Cam for rides while we dined out. When conversation dried up, she'd just gaze in adoration at our only begotten son.

Finally we'd arise and say, “Well, it was nice of you to do this. When will we see you next?” Even then she'd linger in the door or driveway. A couple of times we simply left her standing in the kitchen while Les gave Cam a bath and I disappeared downstairs.

What did she want from us?

We attributed some of her eccentricity to loneliness: she'd left a religious order and reentered the secular world without kids or vocation. We felt sorry for her. Although she had never specified why she'd renounced her vows, she once alluded to some terrible events that had frightened her so much that she'd left the sisterhood. But the story nourished our misgivings: the woman was starting to seem unbalanced.

The final straw came when I asked Sheila to take over for Penny while I went to a meeting. Cam had been slightly under the weather but had no fever and seemed chipper, so I didn't worry. I came home to find Les and Penny sitting on our sofa, looking somber. Sheila was not there.

Apparently she'd been a little too eager to have Cam to herself. "You can leave," she'd urged Penny. "Don't worry, I've handled sick kids quite a bit in my day." Then she'd started riffling through our medicine cabinet looking for a thermometer. Her behavior was bizarre enough that Penny had insisted on calling Les.

"Leslie, Cam is sick."

"Is he getting worse?"

"Well, it's not that. Uh, Sheila thinks we should take his temperature." She whispered, "She's been looking all over for a rectal thermometer. She won't give up. She's acting really weird. I'm afraid to leave."

"I'll be right home."

The next day we told Sheila we had a full complement of therapists and couldn't offer her any work, which was only a white lie: we did have five other therapists to keep busy. But she wasn't about to give up. Perhaps thinking I was the easier mark, she began appearing right after school, saying things like, "You look really tired."

She'd pretend to address Cam. "Cameron, your dad needs a break. Shall we go for a ride?" I'd stammer out some excuse—anything to keep them in my sight.

Then, without warning, she vanished: no call, no explanation, nothing. It seemed strange that she hadn't at least bade Cam goodbye, but we didn't question our good fortune.

A few months later we ran into her at the supermarket. During the small talk, she casually mentioned having been hospitalized. The next day she phoned to ask if she could bring Cam to visit her family. My wife hung fire for a few seconds, then said, "I don't think so. You know how Cam is with new people."

"They really like handicapped kids. My two brothers have MS, you know."

"Well, Sheila, where do your folks live?"

"Oh, down in Florida."

Les's mouth flew open; she looked at me and shook her head. "Sheila, I don't think that would be a good idea. Can you picture Cam on a plane?"

"A plane?" I said.

"Oh, I could handle him. I've dealt with just about everything, believe me. I'd give him lots to do—puzzles, music, and stuff. He might even think it was fun." She offered this lunatic notion in total seriousness.

Only after we finally got her to hang up did astonishment give way to fear. All that pandering, those risky trips, and that constant hovering now took on a sinister cast. Had she harbored this plan all along, the car rides a ploy to accustom Cameron to longer and longer journeys?

Cam had inspired Sharon to feats of bravery, but he'd awakened the darker side of Sheila. Ironically, the fact that he gave back so little emotionally had incited ever more desperate schemes to win his love and salve her fear of abandonment.

The experience left a residue of guilt. How could we have made such an error? What if someone else—someone more devious—managed to worm her way into our lives? Was our carefully designed therapy program putting our child in danger? Was it really worth the risk?

We decided it was, for by mid-1996 our son had made remarkable progress: his working memory had improved, his attention span had lengthened, and his tolerance for work had increased. His imitation and receptive language abilities were vastly better. The five-year-old who couldn't put a single piece into a puzzle could now complete a twelve-piece puzzle on his own.

Hope, that thing with feathers, had dipped and veered, but it had never crashed, for we had stayed focused on the ultimate prize: recovery. We kept our ears tuned, believing that the hidden self perching inside our son would soon start singing his own bright song.

Chapter 7

Melting Down

And so the babe grew up a pretty boy,
A pretty boy, but most unteachable—
And never learn'd a prayer, or told a bead
... But whistled, as he were a bird himself.
—Coleridge, "The Foster Mother's Tale"

Premonitions

I sit reviewing Cam's school notebook. It's only November (1996), but something has already gone badly wrong. On the second day of school, his teacher, Mrs. Minter, reported that Cam was having "major allergy issues" that were causing him to sneeze compulsively and bite his hands. Wasn't allergy therapy supposed to remedy these problems? Last year Cam wore a piece of rubber surgical tubing that gave him something to bite on besides his schedule cards or his neighbor. Now he is chomping down so hard that he has destroyed the tubing.

During library visits, he refuses to sit in a circle and listen to a story he can't follow, knowing if he grabs one of the other kids he'll be removed from the group. Only a week into the semester, Leslie had written to Mrs. M: "We sure don't want to revisit [the final year with Mrs. DeMazio] when Cam ended up isolated, anxious, and aggressive (what a charming combination!). He *desperately* wants to sing songs and do circle activities. I'm guessing that he feels the other kids are preventing this and he is striking out."

By late September, he stopped talking and sleeping. One October day he peed at school five times, not once in the toilet. Yet this is the same classroom, the same teacher, and many of the same classmates he had last year, when Mrs. Minter adopted our Lovaas drills for Cam's curriculum and he had his most successful academic term.

One classmate bawls inconsolably every time someone opens a door. Cam reacts by pulling his hair and hitting anyone within reach. Does the crying bother Cam's ears? Is the pace too rapid? Are the lights too bright?

Hoping to discover the reason and forestall a catastrophe, I've set up a visit to school.

Incarceration

The visit was a disaster. My son acted as though he'd rather hurt himself than be in this classroom with these people. Confused, rattled, and anxious, he couldn't work, though he showed remarkable persistence and ingenuity in tearing his classmates' shirts and snatching his aide's hair. Every time he raised a hand or growled, his aide (a stocky, fortyish woman named Wanda) or teacher would look at him and say, "Cameron, no," or move his hand. He was getting abundant attention for being the black sheep of the flock. Not surprisingly, he stayed in character.

I tried to sit unobtrusively in the corner, but every two minutes Cam peeked at me, frowned, and grabbed the person next to him. As the day degenerated, I tried to give tips, engage Cam's attention, show the staff how to work with him, but with each intervention Cam grew more anxious. I should have sat silently, but it's hard to keep still when you see your child suffering.

The worst moment came when the group left for art class. In the hallway, Cam suddenly dropped to his knees, lay down on the mud-colored floor, and began kicking at the air as if daring Wanda to approach. When coaxing failed, she tried to pick him up. My son snarled and clawed at her shirt. When she dodged and grabbed his hands, he head-butted her chest.

"Just leave him there and walk away. He'll probably get up before long," I advised. It seemed obvious that Cam *wanted* her to try to pick him up so he could vent his rage at her. She backed off, but he was too far gone: instead of getting up, he wailed more loudly. Kids from other classes had begun filling the corridor; we couldn't leave him lying there and thrashing around, so Wanda again tried to pull him to his feet. Cam responded with the intensity and focus of the athlete that, in another life, he might have been: darting at her, he clamped his teeth into her forearm.

"Cameron! Stop!" she shouted.

"Cam, let go right now!" I pulled his head back until he let go. Screaming, he sprawled backward onto the floor. I yanked the squirming boy to his feet, threw him over my back like a bag of grain and lugged him back to the classroom. Wanda followed, tears streaming down her cheeks.

Breathing heavily, I set Cam down. As Wanda and I dropped dejectedly into plastic chairs, Cam clapped, shouted, and nervously roamed the deserted room. "I'm so sorry. I don't know what gets into him," I said.

She choked out, "He hasn't done *that* before. Wow!"

We sat mutely for several minutes. I felt like crying. Though furious and appalled at Cam's behavior, I was just as angry at the staff who'd let this happen and at myself for not doing something sooner.

At home, I brooded bluely over what I'd witnessed. As I skimmed the readings for my next day's classes, the characters, with their romantic problems and confrontations with authority, seemed unimaginably banal, their creators' artfully crafted words worthless. What good was literature—what good was education—when it gave me no tools to help my son? My eyes drifted to the photos of Cam as a toddler: there he was in his bright orange outfit, "Spot" books scattered at his feet, gleefully clapping his chubby hands. There he was a few months later, smiling broadly, bedecked in blue and white overalls. How had this adorable baby turned into the miserable, aggressive child I'd seen at school?

The teacher wrote home that evening, "Cam's anxiety this morning was amazing to me, but understandable. Rule #1: Parents do not belong in school (his rule), just like Cam became anxious when I entered his home. #2: he had conflicts with directions/procedures coming from too many places. #3: too many people were too close."

Translation: I was to blame. It was true. Despite my good intentions, I'd only helped trigger an explosion.

Over the next few weeks, Cam's moods continued to swing wildly: one minute he was giddy with laughter, and the next he'd be crying, slapping his chest, or gnawing on his shirt. Tiny changes or setbacks he once accepted with equanimity sent him into rages. And his bad school days were now spilling over into Lovaas sessions.

We suspected that frustrated intelligence was fueling his fury, an idea borne out at that fall's Lovaas update workshop. Les mentioned in passing that Cam would no longer touch the finger paints he'd briefly enjoyed. As the discussion continued, the crew lost track of Cam for a few minutes. When Les went to fetch him, she found a boy whose complexion had miraculously changed from pink to blue. Evidently the mention of finger paints had inspired Cam, who had smeared himself head to foot—as well as the floor, tabletop, and closet—with blue paint.

Leslie barely remembered where the paints were stored. But not only did Cam remember where they were, he'd also figured out how to get them down from the top shelf of his closet.

The crew laughingly cleaned up the mess. But the rest of the workshop was less merry, especially when Diane Ellison got a taste of what the therapists had been reporting since September. After Cam grabbed her hair and repeatedly slapped her, she told us we couldn't continue under these circumstances and urged us to suspend the program temporarily.

Although we agreed, I felt despondent. The program had given us some control over our son's education, which was otherwise falling apart. Suspending the program felt to me like giving up, giving in to the autism demon. Our belief that Cam knew more than he could express made this development all the more painful.

It felt like a low point. But it wasn't the nadir. We actually hit bottom not long after, a night that is indelibly etched on my memory. Cam had arrived home from school upset but had settled down to complete his work session. We had an appointment with our financial advisor that evening, so Les was giving him an early bath. All of a sudden Cam began to kick violently and emit ear-piercing screams.

What was wrong this time? I could barely care. By now the stress had become unbearable: not only was school a disaster, but Cam was again waking up most nights, our finances were in disarray, and I was afraid we wouldn't make it to the end of the month. My son's howling, each cry louder than the last, felt like a club bludgeoning my head. As the wails continued, the blood rushed to my face. I simply could not stand this any longer.

After one truly painful shriek, I sprang from my chair and barged into the bathroom. "Cameron! Damn it, shut up!" I grabbed him by the back of his hair and gave him a shake. He yelped in surprise, then resumed bawling, even more loudly than before.

"God damn it, stop that!" I bellowed. I saw my angry red face in the mirror.

Water splashed the floor and walls as Leslie pulled our kicking, screaming son from the tub. Two strands of dark hair clung to her cheek as she snapped her head toward me. "Mark, what are you doing!? Get the hell out of here!"

"I'm not leaving. He needs to stop that shit!"

"He can't stop, you idiot!" Her voice rattled the tiny bathroom's tiled walls. With surprising speed and strength, she shoved me through the door and locked it from the inside.

I pounded on the door. "Leslie! Open the door! Now!"

"I'm not opening the door. You're going to hurt him!"

"No, I'm not!" My voice took on a pleading tone. "Jesus Christ, you can't lock me out of my own bathroom!" I stood fuming silently for ten more seconds and then roared, "Open the fucking door!"

"No!" The frayed edge of her voice cut into my ears. I heard sounds of slipping and grappling as she tried to hold Cam down on the wet floor to prevent him from banging his head.

All of a sudden Cam stopped wailing. "Trapped!" he shouted.

Dead silence.

I fell back against the wall and covered my face in my hands. I had no idea he even knew the word that seemed to sum up his seven years of misery and frustration. Suffering had forced it from his mouth. Now it was all clear: Cameron understood his life, his condition—everything. And we were making it worse.

"Please open the door, hon," I begged. My voice had become a croak.

Steam billowed from the room as the door opened. Cam knelt on the floor in a puddle of water, slapping it with his right hand. My wife, her white T-shirt soaked through, squatted down and hugged him hard, rocking from side to side.

"'Trapped.' That pretty much says it all, doesn't it?" I said. She gazed up at me, her eyes wet with tears.

Cam escaped to his room, but Les and I had nowhere to go. We stood in the narrow hallway, hugging, swaying together, sobbing into each other's hair.

Serious mental impairment carries built-in armor: the person is too disabled to realize that he *is* impaired. We'd thought Cam wore this armor, but he'd proven us wrong.

That night, as I tried to force myself to sleep, I replayed those few minutes over and over. I tried to envision living inside Cam's head. I imagined myself inside a body that wouldn't obey my commands. I wanted to say, "My ears hurt," but couldn't find the words. I was constantly bombarded by chaotic sensations but unable to voice my frustration and fear except by screaming or slapping. I saw others staring at me, mocking me, shunning me. I knew I was different but was helpless to do anything about it. As Leslie breathed evenly beside me, I silently wept again.

Exploration

Matters were coming to a head at school: the mother of one of Cam's classmates threatened to hold her son out of school until our son was removed. She'd even phoned the other parents, trying to mount a boycott to force us out. Timberland's principal, who'd told us of the boycott, suggested we keep Cameron at home until we found another placement.

We couldn't entirely blame the boy's parents—they were only trying to protect their son—and Leslie wrote Mrs. Minter a conciliatory note. But we were furious and indignant. Who the hell did they think they were? Why hadn't they called us first and tried to help? How could they be so callous—weren't we all in the same boat? Nope: *they* were in the boat and we were in the water, drowning.

A few days later Leslie called another mom—a woman with whom she'd been friendly in the past—and pleaded with her not to join the boycott.

"We understand why Mrs. Gibbons is worried about her son. And we're well aware that Cam has serious problems. We *are* looking for another placement . . . ." Her voice cracked.

"Don't worry, honey. We're not going to join the boycott. After all, my kid's got his own issues. I mean, if we do this once, who's next?"

Apparently most of the other parents agreed; they resisted the boycott and we stood firm, hoping to force the county's hand. It worked: the next week, the principal called a team meeting to decide on Cam's placement. Ms. Minter told us that in her seventeen years of teaching she'd never seen the wheels move so quickly.

The Baltimore County officials were no doubt eager to get rid of the kid who was fouling up their prized pilot program and raising havoc with other parents. They offered no objection to our leaving the county school system.

But where else could Cam go?

In December we began the search. The first stop, Oakmont, was state-of-the-art—an Ivy League elementary school for the developmentally disabled. Every kid in the eleven- to thirteen-year-old class was even given a laptop computer (this was in 1996, long before laptops became ubiquitous)! We saw a lot of happy and industrious children and quite a few who seemed on the same level as Cam.

But Oakmont was a good hour's drive from our house through the chronically congested Washington-area traffic. That meant at least two hours every day when Cam would be supervised by unqualified people—two hours when he'd have no place to pee. And though the school staff, mostly middle-aged and older women, seemed competent, we doubted they could handle our anxious, hyperaggressive son. Oakmont didn't seem a likely prospect.

The next week we visited Parkview School, housed in a huge tumbledown Victorian mansion, complete with winding staircases and high ceilings. The grounds were well kept, with a playground and field—although nobody was playing there—and a dormitory next door. The director, a harried-looking woman in her forties, was friendly but guarded. We soon found out why.

The contrast with Oakmont was stark: this was a bunch of kids in a warehouse. In the sole classroom, allegedly "higher-functioning" kids played cards.

In another room, a girl of nine or ten lay on a bench, thumbing through a magazine with no apparent comprehension. In the "gym" (a living room containing a large plastic climber), another girl sat smiling and rocking, oblivious to her tangled hair and smudged face. When Les spoke to her, she answered with loud wails: she obviously understood what was being said—something about Christmas and Santa Claus—but had no way of communicating: no pictures, no device, nothing. And why hadn't somebody at least bothered to brush her hair? Another boy ran wildly around the room, stopping every fifteen seconds to switch off the lights, which the aide who patiently trailed him flicked back on. Lights off, lights on—an endless circuit. Didn't they have anything else for him to do?

At the dorms we met Melvin, a chubby African American teenager, who gave a friendly smile, shook hands, and began to ask questions.

"Do you have a dog at your house? Do you have a cat? Do you have a basement? Does it have carpet? Do you have music tapes? Boyz II Men, 'End of the Road?'" Melvin didn't wait for answers because he didn't care about them: the questions were a tape *he* was playing—another endless circuit.

He started through his litany again, "Do you have a dog? Do you have a cat?"

I tried to answer. "Yes, I have a whole bunch of music tapes. I don't have 'End of the Road,' though."

"End of the Road?" he echoed. "Boyz II Men. Do you have it?"

"No, I don't have that one."

"Do you have a basement?"

"I have a basement. It's where I work."

"Does it have carpet?"

The director intervened: "Okay, Melvin, that's enough." To us: "He asks everybody the same questions." As Melvin's aide came to take him elsewhere, Melvin asked, "Can I have a hug?" I was ready to oblige, but the director stepped between us, discreetly noting that Melvin lacked "an appropriate sense of how hard to hug" and when to let go. Though I felt little guilty that I'd denied Melvin some human contact, I was thankful I hadn't been crushed by his friendly embrace.

Despite Melvin's charm, we departed from Parkview with a shudder. The staffers seemed kind and some of the kids may have had potential, but nothing was being done for them. The place was right out of some Gothic novel.

"I'll quit my job and keep Cam home before I send him there," Les said firmly. Amen.

Last on our list was the Callaway Carver School, associated with the well-known Callaway Carver Institute. This was more like what we'd had in mind: children like Cam, a knowledgeable staff and supervisors, and an entire hospital full of experts nearby to consult if need be. The principal, Martha Lawrence,

EdD, a brisk, square-jawed woman with the bluff mien of a football coach, ran a tight ship. Clearly nobody gave her any grief.

They had no opening.

Education

Cam's days at Timberland did not improve. Ms. Minter wrote home, "I don't know what will happen now. We are trying to involve Cam in all our Xmas activities—songs, projects, etc., but he becomes agitated and says 'all done' frequently. Even when projects are done one-to-one he fights during them."

We'd asked her in a previous note if Cam might be bored, reasoning that boredom might prompt his antisocial behavior. She answered,

I'm sure he is slightly bored—he's not able to participate in most of our activities or chooses not to. Walks have been disasters—tantrums on most of them. He chooses his own space isolated from the others on many occasions. We created new tasks and he chewed or tore up the materials. Even his individualized schedule seems to be not what he needs.

This is a teacher at the end of her rope. She just wants the boy to go away.

Hoping an objective assessment would make that happen, we tried to call in Katherine Clifton, a specialist at the Callaway Carver Autism Center. But for some reason the Timberland officials resisted the visit, and when they finally yielded, Dr. Clifton was unavailable for several more weeks.

When at last we managed to get her to our house for a visit and assessment, she watched Cam at dinner and in one of the play sessions that had replaced Lovaas/ABA therapy. Naturally, he showed off for her, so she witnessed none of the aggression they complained about at school. Later she visited Cam's classroom twice, and sent a letter to all concerned.

It is a sobering assessment. First she notes that Cameron did not respond well to the "visual structure of the classroom and the rapid pace of activities and transitions," and that his classmates' distracting behaviors have "become overwhelming for him. Thus, he has become resistant to almost all demand-oriented activities."

She continues,

he engages in a . . . repertoire of behaviors as soon as he . . . perceives certain cues. One of those cues is literally the front door of Timberland Elementary School. Another cue is the presence of the assistant in Mrs. M's classroom—he demonstrates a much higher rate of problematic behavior in her presence. . . . This suggests that most of his inappropriate behavior serves the functions of escape.

She verified our belief that Cam hated the place and everybody in it. No doubt they didn't care for him either. A boy who pulls your hair, throws himself to the floor, wails, and demands constant attention: who could like such a frightening blend of bully and baby?

Dr. Clifton's next words confirmed our other suspicions: "Cameron has likely gained an incredible amount of reinforcement for his inappropriate behaviors, simply via the natural reactions of the other students and adults . . . and he is certainly sharp enough to recognize a desired reaction when he gets it." In other words, Cam had learned the black sheep's lesson: everyone looks at me when I'm bad.

Dr. Clifton advised us to start over—above all, to find a new school immediately—honor appropriate communication, reintroduce work sessions gradually, and replace bad behaviors with good ones. Unfortunately, she warned, Cam had been heading down the wrong path for so long that it would be difficult to turn him around; his nasty behaviors were now firmly established coping tactics. Like a veteran who still thinks he's at the front and responds to every "hello" with a thrusting bayonet, Cam's trauma had turned tendencies into inflexible patterns, sweeping away his personality and leaving in its wake a collection of destructive habits and ingrown fetishes.

The report marked another turning point in our life with autism. I thought back to Cam at age two, when he'd taken the first detour off the road of typical development, and recalled our gradual recognition that something scary was taking place. I felt the same helplessness, fear, and isolation wash over me once again. But if it was difficult for us, it was infinitely worse for our son: his disorder was hardening around him like a carapace; the more desperately he struggled, the more tightly it clutched him.

Explosion

One therapy that still worked was weekly horse-riding lessons. Cam loved Oreo, the mild-mannered pony he rode, and proudly crowed when astride him. The lessons calmed him down, gave him a sense of purpose, and provided structure for our aimless Saturdays.

One Saturday that winter, I drove Sam to a convention in Washington, DC, leaving Les with our battered, rusty 1980 Corolla—the one with no rear seat belts. It wasn't a good car for Cam, since he had to ride in the front, where he had access to the driver, stick shift, and dashboard, but we'd forgotten that Les would have to drive Cam to his riding lesson that day.

I returned to find a traumatized wife. She couldn't even talk about what had happened but kept saying, "I did something terrible. Terrible. I don't know what's wrong with me. I abused my own child."

I tried to console her. "Oh, hon, I doubt that. You don't even spank him!"

"I did. I'll never forgive myself." Her dark eyes were opaque.

Several days later she finally told the story. The riding lesson had gone well. But as they approached the beltway exit that leads to our neighborhood, Cam—for no apparent reason—started throwing himself against the seat. Seconds later he was slapping at her hands and pulling her hair. She gamely tried to ward off the attacks while keeping the car on the road.

Why didn't they just pull over? They were so close to home that Les thought it made more sense to keep driving. Then Cam grabbed the steering wheel. The car swerved toward the median, and Les was barely able to wrench the wheel away and force the car back on course before it crashed.

For one of the few times in our life with autism, my wife truly lost her temper. "Stop it! Stop! Stop! Stop!" she screamed, slapping Cam on the top of the head and back of the neck.

Shocked—Mommy never blew up like this—Cam shrank away, then started wailing.

What was he trying to say? That he didn't want to ride this far? That he wanted me there? That he had to pee? A couple of months later, Les arrived at this hypothesis: she'd been driving the wrong car. In Cam's mind, the brown car was Daddy's car, and Mommy shouldn't drive Daddy's car. Cam's cup of anxiety was so near the brim that this small change had made it overflow. On that day, switching cars was an unforgivable crime.

I didn't blame Les for losing her cool but couldn't stop her from blaming herself: "I don't know what got into me. It was wrong, wrong, wrong." I doubt Cam even remembers it. Yet for years afterward she obsessed over this incident, inflating it into a criminal case of child abuse. I'd tell her that most people would have blown their top sooner and more often—as, indeed, I had done many times. Yet I also know that her rage wasn't really directed at Cam: it was aimed at the other passenger in the car, the one who made him bite his aide and throw a tantrum in the bathtub. She was angry at autism itself, which seemed to have an unending supply of ways to torture us.

Medication

We couldn't wait for a new school; we had to do something immediately. Dr. Archer recommended that we consult a neurologist at CC Institute.

An affable fellow in his forties, Dr. Arthur Frank resembled the comic actor Gene Wilder, and his slightly crooked smile and wild, curly hair put us at ease. For three-quarters of an hour, he listened compassionately to our tale of woe. Meanwhile, the protagonist sat giggling and humming to himself.

I gestured at our placid son. "This is the boy who can't sit still at school. Can you see why we think a good share of this is a result of the school situation?"

"Yes," the doctor agreed. "He gets so anxious and upset at school that he can't calm himself afterwards. But when the environment is relaxed, he can relax."

As if on cue (had he understood?), Cam rose and moved the chair to the examination pallet. He climbed up, then climbed down; up, down, up, down. He scrutinized the paper, wadded it up, chewed it. He moved the chairs to the sofa and tried to stack them; when the chairs inevitably toppled over, he restacked them. The doctor watched him carefully, then chuckled.

"He's quite the little planner. I'd say there's a good deal of potential there."

We were thankful for his words, and even more thankful when he wrote a prescription for a drug called Klonopin: "It's designed to reduce his anxiety. We'll start with a small dose, then work our way up. Come back in a week and let me know how he's doing."

As we left his office, the world looked a little brighter: an expert had told us our son wasn't hopeless and even seemed confident he could help him.

But the results were ambiguous. Cam seemed less anxious, but his eyes looked glassy. And he couldn't sit for more than a minute, even during meals. School days seemed to be going a little better, but it wasn't clear whether the improvement was a result of the drug or of the kinder aide who'd replaced Wanda (she'd quit: who could blame her?). Again we saw what we wanted to see—that the medication was helping Cam concentrate and relax—so we kept him on it through the winter.

Then, one morning during spring break in 1997, I noticed a large welt running across Cam's back. Further inspection revealed more hives. Over the next hour they moved to his arms, fingers, and legs, before gradually fading away.

I called Leslie at work, then phoned Cam's allergist. He advised us to give Cam his medication as usual and watch closely to see if the hives came back. They did. I brought Cameron to see him that afternoon.

Although he'd been prescribing allergy treatments for a year, this was the first time the doctor had examined the boy in person. A soft-spoken fellow in his mid-fifties, Dr. Payton sported an oddly regular hairline. After a few minutes of covert peeks, I realized he had plug transplants. "Great," I thought, "our doctor is Elton John." Suddenly I no longer trusted him.

Allergies were the order of the day, all right: the doctor seemed to be allergic to his patient, whom he examined gingerly, as if he exuded a foul smell.

"Those are some pretty big hives. Has he ever had them before?"

"No. They were going away, but they came back right after I gave him his second dose of Klonopin."

"These enormous hives are a bad sign. We might not get any more warning, and then one day he could go into anaphylactic shock, which could be fatal. You need to call the doctor who prescribed the drug and tell him what's going on. In the meantime, don't give him any more of the medication."

On our way out, the doctor confided, "I wish the parents who come here and complain about their kids could have been with us today. They'd see how lucky they are." I was too rattled to feel insulted.

Dr. Frank seemed unperturbed, though he agreed that we should take Cam off the drug. He cautioned us, "We don't like to cut off a drug like Klonopin abruptly, because he might have some withdrawal symptoms."

"Such as what?" I asked, recalling horror stories about junkies kicking the habit.

"Probably some difficulty sleeping, maybe some problems with body temperature and mood swings."

Those didn't sound too terrible, since Cam experienced two of the three already. So we weren't prepared for what followed. As the drug wore off, Cam's body craved it. His mood swings grew violent: without warning he'd growl, then fall to the floor in a tantrum; minutes later he couldn't keep his eyes open. For several days, he took long midday naps; he'd fall asleep those nights but wake at 2 a.m., his little body covered with sweat. He had spells of uncontrollable shivering, as if standing outdoors coatless in the dead of winter.

Our seven-year-old was going cold turkey.

We were worried; but more than that we felt ashamed for putting our child through this agony. On top of his problems with school, his failing Lovaas program and toilet training regression, he now had to cope with a drug addiction. It was too much. One day Cam came home from school, lay on the couch, and cried and cried—the hopeless sobbing of a child whose body has betrayed him. After two weeks, Cam returned to his old self. We swore we'd never again put him on a drug.

At the next visit Dr. Frank told us that night sweats, shaking, mood swings, insomnia, and hyperactivity were all part of "normal withdrawal from the drug." Easy for him to say. As we prepared to leave, he said, "I'm conducting an experiment, and I wonder if you guys want to take part. Here's how it goes. We take spinal taps to see if the spinal fluid of autistic children is chemically different from those of other kids. This is important research because it might provide a basis for better analyses of their brains and the chemistry of their central nervous systems."

He proposed this so calmly and affably that we actually considered it for a moment. But by the time we'd returned home we were furious. While we'd been describing our son's season in hell, the doctor who'd helped to put him there was thinking about his next research project. To him Cam was not a suffering kid; he was a guinea pig.

Worst of all was our belated realization that Cam's behavior was no different now than it had been while on the Klonopin. We'd put him through all this for nothing.

Notification

Relief finally arrived in late February, when Callaway Carver School notified us that they were accepting Cam for a ten-day trial period, beginning in early April. The only potential pitfall was his biting: because bites spread diseases, Dr. Lawrence warned, it was one of the few behaviors that could eliminate him. But we barely heard her: we had glimpsed the promised land.

Ms. Minter was equally relieved. "Yay!" she wrote home. "I can hang on for a few more weeks!" Those weeks passed in a blur.

Finally, on April 15, 1997, Cameron started at CC. After dropping him off that first day, I walked to the car feeling like Noah after the flood. Cam shared the feeling: we suddenly had a happy child again.

Still, the probation period wore on us. Cam seemed worried: he couldn't sleep and began to gnaw habitually on his hands. We anxiously read the notes from school. For each positive message—"Cameron sat calmly with the group during circle time, and worked well at his cubicle this afternoon"—there was another one like this: "Cameron couldn't work at all after lunch." His teacher had remarked on how cute he was, and we clung to that positive sign.

At last, on the eleventh day, Dr. Lawrence called to tell us that Cam had been accepted. We were beyond feeling exultant; mostly we felt dazed. We told Cam he had passed the audition. The next day he bit his aide.

Chapter 8

Holding Patterns

A fiery soul, which working out its way
Fretted the pigmy body to decay:
And o'er inform'd the tenement of clay
A daring pilot in extremity . . .
—John Dryden, "Absalom and Achitophel"

Pilots in Extremity

Cam is working. Or rather, his therapist is—Cam is more interested in rocking in his chair. *Baaaack,* then *clunk. Baaack* and *clunk. Baaaaacccckkk* and *clunk!*

"No," she admonishes. "It's learning time. Put with same."

"No, okay!" He grabs the cardboard letter and thrusts it into his mouth, then springs from the chair and throws himself on the bed.

In mid-1997, we revived the Lovaas program, patching together a crew of aides from Cam's school, the daughter of Les's boss (a psychology major), and two new hires.

Cam loved his new voice output device, which helped him say what he wanted to say. And he was so fascinated with coins that we began to use them as rewards. But he didn't seem to understand the concept of numbers and still couldn't handle a crayon or pencil. He memorized the QWERTY keyboard but couldn't use the letters to make words. In short, all three R's remained beyond his ken.

Diane Ellison might have helped, but she wasn't available. That fall we scheduled two update workshops and she missed both, giving weak excuses each time. Had she lost interest in Cam?

To prepare for the workshop in May 1998, she asked us to videotape Cam's sessions so she could evaluate his progress and determine how to update the program. The tapes dramatized the clever avoidance tactics our son had devised. Gone were the days when he'd softly say "potty" or break into song. Now he began most sessions with a loud request to "go ahead" (the prompt to end the session).

"No, Cam. We have to work now."

He'd slap the table and rock in the chair. "Go 'head!"

"No. It's learning time."

Out would come his hands, reaching for the therapist's shirt.

"Hands down."

"Go 'head!" Red-faced, nearly shouting.

Sometimes he'd wrap himself in blankets and refuse to come out (we learned to strip the bed before sessions). He'd feign fascination with a thread in his shirt or a stray piece of paper, then shove the paper into his mouth or up his nostril. He'd have giggling fits or clap his hands frantically and guffaw.

Other tactics were more overtly antagonistic. He so often destroyed the matching cards that we had to laminate them, and they still looked like they'd been attacked by teething puppies. The cardboard puzzles also took a beating: frustrated at having to start over, or mad that he couldn't wedge a piece into the wrong place, Cam would chew the offending fragment. The misshapen pieces only made his task harder. The riskiest drill was nonverbal imitation, which required the therapist to sit knee-to-knee with Cam, putting hair and arms within reach of his grabbing hands. If all else failed, he'd pee on the floor.

When I intervened, I sometimes managed to settle him down (with a rapid-fire imitation drill) and let the therapist continue; other days, I'd allow a snack or TV break. More often, Cam would simply direct his fury at me—slapping, scratching, pinching, yanking on my shirt. If none of that worked, he'd try the tactic of last resort: biting. By then, there was no point in continuing the session. I often left the room sweating, my bloody hands fingering a torn shirt.

We tried never to end after aggression. But sometimes just closing the door to start a session brought slaps. He was so adept at finding ways of avoiding work: why couldn't he use that intelligence productively?

We wondered if the bad sessions were carryovers from school, but couldn't find a pattern: uneventful school days were often paired with terrible home sessions; other days showed the opposite trend. Strangely, during good sessions—about half the time—he worked as well as ever.

Cam's preferences were also unpredictable: one week he liked playing racquetball and the next he would only gnaw on the ball; for two weeks he enjoyed using crayons and then decided to eat them. One thing was consistent—aggression. It had become what he did during sessions: "I delay, they coax, I act up, but we keep going until I blow up and Daddy comes." Aggression had become an autistic habit, an unstoppable train running on its circular track.

Our therapists didn't quit. Why? Because, despite the hitting and the hair pulling, the bloody knuckles and the frightening rages, they sensed a child struggling to emerge and sometimes caught a glimpse of him: the boy who kissed their cheeks and cooed, who laughed when they laughed, who concentrated so hard that he'd bring tears to their eyes—a boy who, beneath the bizarre and irritating behavior, needed and wanted their help.

What was Cam trying to tell us? That there were too many people in his life—too many therapists, teachers, kids? That we were working him too hard? We *were* expecting a lot from him: full school days followed by two-hour sessions at home, plus one or two sessions on weekends. We were asking him to gather his scattered attention, communicate, think in sequence—the very skills he found most difficult.

Whatever he was saying, Diane Ellison didn't like it. The night before the scheduled May workshop, she phoned us.

"My supervisor and I watched those videotapes you sent."

"Yeah? What did you think?"

"His aggression is completely out of hand."

"He's had some lousy sessions lately. But he's also had some good ones. He's moving along pretty well on quite a few of the drills. The typing is going great, and he really likes the coins."

"Maybe so. But we have to think about everybody's safety. You can't keep asking therapists to subject themselves to that kind of treatment. We're on the verge of somebody getting hurt."

"They're all really tolerant. I talk to them a lot, and they don't get upset."

"It's not just that. Even when Cameron isn't aggressive, he's not compliant. I saw a *lot* of stimming. All that clapping and chest beating and avoidance. Having to coax him to come to the table. And when he gets there he doesn't pay attention half the time. All that stuff goes against the whole idea of the program. We have to question whether it's doing what it's supposed to do."

I had nothing to say. Where was this going?

"We've seen this before. When these kids start getting older, if they're not making the kind of progress that's going to get them mainstreamed, they start to rebel. It's a lot of pressure, you know, to do discrete trials for years and years."

"Too much repetition?"

"Partly that. It's more that they start to rebel against being confined and the whole method of rewards. How old is Cameron now?"

"Almost nine."

"That's just about the time. You can drill, drill, drill a three- or four- or five-year-old. But when they get to be seven or eight it gets harder and harder. The kids want to have more say. They start rejecting the reinforcers and act like you're bribing them."

"So what does this mean?" I heard my voice getting husky.

"I think we need to stop following a straight academic program and move to a less-structured approach."

I didn't like the sound of this. "Like what?"

"We recommend moving back to structured play sessions along with scheduled outings. Kind of like we did last year."

I didn't want to hear it; stopping the program again was unthinkable. We decided to go ahead with the workshop while Les and I thought it over. I spent the night fuming: they were abandoning us, they weren't seeing the good side, Cam had been doing better lately, and so on.

The next day Diane stuck to her guns: abandon ABA and set up a schedule of outings to the park, the store, and such. Establish play skills such as swinging, riding the bike, and playing ball. The more she talked about it, the more plausible it seemed. The therapists were clearly relieved: these sessions' modest demands wouldn't incite the kind of punishment Cam had been meting out.

I had no choice but to go along. Even I realized that the program needed a makeover: many drills had gone stale, and Cam resisted even ones he used to like. Yet inwardly I rebelled. My feelings were partly selfish: I'd have to monitor the therapists more closely than I had been. Les's work schedule was so demanding that she barely had the energy to give Cam an evening bath, let alone spend weekends devising a curriculum. That meant setting up the program, thinking of ideas and following through with them, would fall mostly to me. I didn't mind the work; it was the lack of a clear goal that bothered me. I couldn't face the prospect of losing the structure and consistency the Lovaas sessions gave us—gave me and Les, as much as Cam.

After the workshop, a therapist stayed with Cam while Les and I dined out. I complained that Diane wanted nothing to do with any kid who wouldn't make her program look good; the school was cutting us loose before we dragged down their precious success ratios. But Leslie agreed with Diane: we couldn't continue to ask these girls to get their hair pulled and shirts ripped day after day. When I disagreed, she jolted me with harsh words: "He's mentally retarded, Mark. That's what she's saying. You need to deal with that."

"I can accept that," I lied. "What I can't accept is the way they did this. Not even twenty-four hours' notice! What the hell has Diane been doing for the last few months? She doesn't say anything for ages, and then the night before the big workshop, when we've gone to all this trouble to set everything up, she drops this bomb on us. You know as well as I do that we're going to be stuck with hours of empty time. Cam will get bored, and all hell will break loose."

My protests were camouflage. Since the start of the Lovaas program we'd kept our eyes on the prize—Cam would overcome autism, or at least learn to play, do math, read, write, and talk. But now Diane was telling us that Cam would never catch up—worse, he wouldn't become much more capable than he already was. She was telling us our son would never be a regular kid.

That night I sat in the den, my eyes glued to *Atlantic Monthly,* scanning the same sentences over and over, enveloped in gloom. If Cam couldn't learn to read and write, what kind of life would he have? If he couldn't learn to speak better, how would he tell anybody what he needed? If he couldn't control his rage, where would he go to school, and where would he live as an adult? My son was doomed to lifelong disability. I couldn't accept it. Abandoning the Lovaas program meant that I couldn't *make* Cam get better just by trying harder.

So far in my life, whenever I set a goal, I never gave up until I achieved it. But now I was being asked to give up on my son, who wasn't even nine years old. Was my whole philosophy of life—that hard work conquers all—a fantasy? And what about my other prized faith, the one I'd clung to tenaciously throughout my life, the belief that intelligence is the truest measure of human value? If my beloved son was retarded, then either he was worthless or my life had been based on a lie. To admit that Cam would never be normal was to accept fallibility—my fallibility. It was to admit that *I* was, in some sense, disabled.

I'd been living in Wonderland, and it was time to wake up.

Playing It by Ear

Les and I dutifully set up the new system. One key element was the Language Master machine, which records words on cards and plays them back. We recorded phrases identifying various places, velcroed Polaroids to the cards and put them into a book labeled "Places to Go." Cam would page through the book, choose a photo and card, slide it through the machine, and a voice (mine or Les's) would say, for example, "Playground." Cam would repeat, "Playground, yes," and we'd get going. But he chose the same places every day, and soon got bored with them. Then he'd lapse back into stims: pulling strings from clothes, snapping off tree limbs, compulsively overeating.

Were we supposed to build from the simple to the sophisticated? Should we vary them daily? What was the ultimate goal?

I called Diane frequently to ask these questions, but she was never available. Les and I agreed that Cam craved the attention and sense of competence that discrete-trial sessions had given him. And so, in July we eased back into a modified ABA program, reintroducing Cam's favorite drills and adding some functional and play programs. Using the Language Master, we encouraged him to choose activities outdoors or at least outside his room.

We were flying by the seat of the pants—without a pilot's license. We groped along, guided by our therapists' experiences and those of the overtaxed staff at Cam's school. I copied some drills from Catherine Maurice's *Let Me Hear Your Voice* and asked other parents about their programs. Sometimes I just made things up.

Jazz musicians follow this rule: if you don't know the harmonies, trust your ears. But successful improvising requires years of training, and I was no special educator; I was a novice musician playing an unknown tune with unfamiliar musicians. What was the next note? How did you know when to stop? How did you all work together?

No doubt we were trying to prove that we hadn't given up, that we were doing all we could. Guilt drove us on: the fear that we'd look back someday and feel we hadn't tried everything possible to help our son. But we did modify our expectations. Where we'd once hoped for a breakthrough, we now aimed for gradual progress. And we forged on.

I still clung to the hope that Cam would someday learn to read. After all, he'd been able to recognize some words when he was a toddler. How could he lose that skill entirely?

For a year, Cam had been matching the letters in his first name to a template. We'd slowly faded the template letters in reverse order, hoping he'd eventually learn to spell "Cameron." With only two or three to choose from, he could usually do it. But when he had to pick the right letters from a stack, Cam stalled, chewed the cards, slapped the table, and gave up. He wasn't misbehaving; he didn't know what the letters meant.

We tried another tactic. He'd already mastered letter-matching and word-matching drills and could even match words to pictures. The next—most crucial—step was to match a word ("sock" or "ball") to the proper object. But the lettered cards baffled Cam: what did this paper thing have to do with a sock or ball? After some random guesses, he'd look helplessly at the therapist. There was no way to offer a hint without giving the answer away. He tried—oh, how he tried. His brows would furrow up and he'd chew on his shirt, concentrating as hard as he could. But he simply could not make the connection. It was heartbreaking. He was trying to play by ear, but his instrument didn't work.

The abstract ideas that a collection of letters represents sounds (phonemes), that a written word represents an object or action, simply eluded him. He could understand that a drawing of someone eating stood for the idea of eating. But real language involves arbitrary links between sounds and concepts or objects: the only reason we connect the sound of the word "dog" to the animal or the shape and letters of the word "sink" to the bathroom fixture is that we're taught to do so. No matter how you learn to read, at some point you must make the cognitive leap that these letter shapes are symbolic. Cam couldn't make the leap; he was frozen in midair.

He was telling us he couldn't do it, but I couldn't hear his message. Reading was itself a symbol for me. If Cam could learn to read, then he wasn't "really" disabled: he was one of us.

The Hatter's Clock

Although Cam maintained his level of competence in most areas, there were maddening instances when he lost a skill or when his fixations interfered. Such was the case with his tape deck. Through long months of repetition, we'd taught him to operate a Fisher-Price cassette player. He could insert and eject tapes, fast-forward and rewind to find his favorite songs. Listening to him scan through his music as he lay in bed at night, buttons snapping and cassette wheels whirring, we smiled happily at our small victory. Cam was in charge of his own music!

So it was a dark day when he discovered that cassettes contain long, thin pieces of tape, and that, if he pulled on them, the whole tape unraveled. All at once, tapes had nothing to do with music, but were simply ribbons to stretch and shred. He destroyed his Raffi tapes, his *Peter and the Wolf,* his Disney sing-alongs—all within weeks.

He'd wait until we weren't watching, then grab the cassette and yank the tape out, stretching it and strewing it around the room. If one of us caught him, he'd cower under his bedcovers. Over and over I'd explain, "Cam, this is your music. If you pull the tape out, the music will be gone. No more music." He'd stare blankly as if he hadn't heard.

Apparently, the tactile pleasure of stretching the long, thin tape was simply too strong to resist. If he briefly regretted ruining a tape, the next time he saw one, he forgot his remorse. Autism was an imp of perversity driving Cam to destroy the very things that gave him pleasure.

When we replaced tapes with CDs, he no longer wanted to find—or wasn't capable of finding—the songs he liked. Was the new skill too difficult to acquire? Was he depressed by the loss of control? We didn't know. We did know that *we* felt like tapes spinning around, playing the same song over and over until we also snapped.

Cam did succeed admirably at one academic drill: functional language. Hoping to give him tools in case (shudder!) he ever got lost, we laboriously taught him a set of responses to questions such as, "What is your name?" "What is your address?" and "Where do you go to school?" Unfortunately, his enunciation was so poor that even his correct responses were unintelligible to anybody who didn't already know the answer.

"What's your address?"

"Tweeboo." Tweedledee? Tweety bird? Teebook?

Cam has trouble pronouncing consonant clusters: thus he says his name is "Camra Otee." I envisioned burly police officers straining to make out his name, running their thick fingers down the O's in the mammoth Baltimore phone book, then fruitlessly calling everyone whose surname started with "Ot."

We were pleased that Cam memorized several responses, including the answer to "How old are you?" He learned that the answer was "ten," and it took several months of drilling to replace it with "eleven." But that was it; he couldn't hold onto further changes. If you ask him today, "How old are you?" he'll look away, then tentatively mutter, "leben." He'd struggled and struggled to learn that answer, and damn it, he wasn't going to give it up. It almost seemed as if Cam recognized his arrested development and feared growing older.

Our son was like the Mad Hatter's clock, eternally frozen at 6 p.m.

Puzzles

Diane Ellison was right about one thing: Cam didn't break through. His memory held him back. Though he can still recite whole passages from toddler books he memorized at age two, his short-term memory is frustratingly erratic. He can't retain some skills or behaviors and retains others all too well. Unfortunately, the skills he finds most difficult are the so-called pivotal behaviors needed for cognitive development: writing, reading, talking, playing. Anything not rote or rule-bound mystifies him.

One criticism leveled at ABA training is that the kids don't learn to generalize. But this isn't, in my view, a problem with the method; it's a problem with the children. Or at least with our child, who either overgeneralized—giving the same answer to every question ("Who is it?" "Daddy")—or under-generalized, as if every skill or program were novel. He couldn't hold onto patterns that counted and held onto patterns that didn't.

Autism specialists Francesca Happé and Uta Frith theorize that many autists lack "central coherence": when they look at, say, a haystack in a field, they don't see a haystack, let alone a field, but individual strands of hay, each one slightly different. Happé suggests that this "cognitive style" is just one extreme along the spectrum of normal human learning styles. But such a skill is meaningless unless you can place the details into a wider context. That's what Cam can't do. His lack of central coherence isn't just a "style"; it's a severe disability.

This theory does, however, explain a tendency that long confounded me. When assembling a puzzle, Cam didn't see an elephant squirting water at a circus; he saw only a group of irregular colored pieces of gray, brown, or red. And though he gained satisfaction from fitting those pieces into their proper slots, the thrill of discovery that motivates neuro-typical kids—oh, look! It's Dumbo taking a bath!—was absent. No matter how many times he put together a puzzle, he seldom recalled that the orange piece always went in the left corner; instead, he'd follow the same trial-and-error method he'd used the first time he saw the puzzle, attempting over and over to place a knob into a slot where it didn't fit. It was as if each piece were a thing unto itself. Likewise, the different parts of the process—problem solving, creating a picture, matching, recalling which colors belong where, visualizing a whole—were confined to separate cells, unable to communicate with each other.

In this regard, at least, the Autism Society of America's logo—a child inside a puzzle—seems apt. Puzzles, and Cam's method of solving them, seemed to symbolize his disability. Despite his laboriously learned coping strategies and compensations, the world remained for him a collection of discrete shapes. Likewise, to us Cam himself seemed a puzzle with missing pieces—the pivotal, interlocking pieces that held everything together.

In cognition, everything is connected. Because Cam couldn't generalize consistently, he couldn't acquire the skills that would have helped him develop further skills. Because his fine motor skills were poor, he couldn't master the movements needed for writing. Not learning to write impeded his ability to read and vice versa, further slowing his cognitive development. That's autism in a nutshell: an engine generating unending vicious cycles, a plane in a perpetual holding pattern.

Aggression was Cam's distress signal—the sign of a scrambled sensory message, a fear, or some unstoppable train of thought. Every Lovaas session reminded him of his disabilities, yet we kept rubbing his nose in them. Perhaps he realized that the drills were no longer helping him. Or maybe he was telling us that he couldn't be the child we wanted him to be.

Just as the intransigence of Cam's disorder mirrored and magnified the good and bad traits of his therapists—Sharon's persistence and good cheer, Sheila's desperation—it brought out the best and worst in his parents. My determination devolved into obstinacy; Leslie's energy propelled her into chronic fatigue. We tried to mold Cam, but instead he molded us.

My son's frustration was painful to see and excruciating to contemplate: "Why can't I remember this? Why can't I understand what they want? Why are they making me do these drills over and over?" Yet I also know that he often felt proud of his accomplishments in the program, insignificant though they may seem to others. His smiles and claps when he completed a puzzle or recognized his name told us that, for once his life, he felt successful. Those moments of joy and satisfaction shone through the disappointments, expense, headaches, and anxieties. At these moments the pieces fit together seamlessly and the jagged lines disappeared.

But if Cam's successes displayed extraordinary courage and resilience, his "failures" showed a different brand of courage—the fiery soul of a child discovering and defending his nature. For him, just living day to day on our inhospitable planet demands a bravery equal to the boldest astronaut's.

Chapter 9

The Red Queen's Race

"A slow sort of country!" said the [Red] Queen. "Now here, you see, it takes all the running you can do to keep in the same place. If you want to get somewhere else, you must run at least twice as fast as that."
—Lewis Carroll, *Through the Looking-Glass*

Between 1995 and 1997, we'd tried megavitamin and magnesium therapy, allergy therapy, vision therapy, medication. We'd tested Cam's ears and eyes. We'd maintained an ABA program and enrolled him in a TEACCH-style classroom. We'd given him riding lessons, taken him swimming, signed him up for gymnastics. He'd learned some academic skills, could deftly handle a fork, and was fully trained for bowel movements. But his autistic behaviors hadn't abated and his aggression was worse. He still regularly wet his pants and bed, couldn't play a game, had no friends, couldn't hold a rudimentary conversation, couldn't read or write his name.

We were running the Red Queen's race against autism.

We considered "alternative" treatments—special diets, auditory training, therapies such as the Sonrise program—but doubted their effectiveness. Of course, we couldn't be sure. The result was constant second-guessing. With a child like Cam, you can *never* do enough—never relax, never let up, for fear of overlooking the one therapy that might help or even cure him.

But hope is hard to kill, and it returned once more after Cam was finally admitted to Callaway Carver. This Blue Ribbon school had on-site physicians, music therapists, speech therapists, physical therapists—a whole panoply of experts. Surely they'd help him!

Faster, Faster!

That first year, 1997–1998, Cam's teacher was Sherry Petrous, a bright, bubbly educator with lots of good ideas. Optimistic, patient, and smart, she seemed perfect. But wherever Cam went, the looking-glass world went with him, and his honeymoon ended quickly.

The music and movement therapists' reports tell the tale of his first year:

Fall 1997: "Cameron is inconsistent with his behaviors during both music and dance therapy groups. He exhibits increased anxiety and aggression. Cameron continues to need prompting for activities, but when he actively participates in groups he does very well." *When* he participated, which wasn't often. He much preferred bouncing on his chair or destroying materials. When they tried to force him to get involved, he hit or pinched staff or students.

Spring 1998: "Cameron continues to display aggression during music and dance therapy. He does fairly well when he is able to focus." "Very well" has become "fairly well." She is losing the battle.

The speech therapy reports were worse: his "grade" for each objective was marked "objective not addressed." In other words, she spent most of her time fending off Cam's aggression instead of teaching him to speak.

Sherry's tactful notes were no more encouraging. "Super day" meant our son hadn't hit anyone and had completed some of his programs; "not a very good day" meant he'd probably drawn blood by nail-gouging someone's hand.

We kept running, but the scenery didn't change.

The teacher and psychiatrist began hinting that we should put Cam on medication. But we had no desire to repeat the Klonopin ordeal. I dismissed their suggestions in a note so curt that Leslie felt the need to append conciliatory remarks:

Mark's note isn't intended to sound mean. It's just that we have truly been through the mill w/ this child. We absolutely recognize your efforts (herculean, in fact) on Cam's behalf. While we are open to discussing meds, we want to make sure that we're not medicating Cam when some sort of environmental restructuring is the real answer. Medication did not solve the classroom problems last year and, in fact, became yet another problem.

In February 1998 the school tried a new punishment protocol: whenever Cam "exhibited antisocial behavior," he had to insert "compliance pegs" into a board for a set number of minutes. One day I observed Cam during "circle time" and group speech therapy. He watched the speech pathologist circle the table with questions—"Who has the ball? Cameron has the ball!"—then at his turn tapped her on the shoulder just hard enough to count as aggression. He was removed from the group—precisely as he'd wanted. He would rather insert compliance pegs for twenty minutes than endure the speech group. Why couldn't these highly trained educators perceive what seemed so obvious—that Cam was manipulating them?

In one note, Sherry reported that he'd done those pegs for most of the previous day. While performing this boring task, Cam kept saying "no hit," and "no kick Mommy"—scripts he'd learned at home. She added, "'Don't hit Mommy.' That's a funny thing for him to say." We heard the insinuation: was he saying "Don't hit Mommy" or "Don't hit, Mommy?" Connections were being made in the staff's busy minds—"Does he hit others because his parents hit him?"— even though they were well aware that he hit anyone who interfered with his desires.

Les was furious. "The worst part of it is that they don't come right out and say it. They just look at you with that fake innocence."

"That way if you confront them they can just deny it." I shook my head. "You know how it is: when in doubt, blame the parents."

"Especially the mom. As if I don't feel guilty enough."

Clearly, Cam's placement was in danger. We agreed to talk with the school psychiatrist about medication.

Risking Risperdal

Dr. Nigel Cohen, a slim man with thick, unruly brown hair and a clipped, chilly Commonwealth accent, met us in his office and began to explain medications. Though put off by his limp handshake, I had to admit that he seemed knowledgeable. Sherry Petrous was also in the room to furnish support— whether for him or for us wasn't clear.

The doctor then asked questions. "How would you assess Cameron's abilities?" He pronounced our son's name with three syllables. "Do you think Cam-er-on is mentally retarded?"

I answered, "Well, to me the word 'retarded' doesn't fit him. He's so bright-eyed and active. I think of retarded as dull and slow. But clearly there's a cognitive impairment. I mean, it's obvious—he can't learn."

He nodded neutrally. "What are your hopes for his future? Do you want him to go to college? To get married?"

I thought for a moment. "At one time we might have, but now we're more realistic. I'd just like him to find one thing to do that will make him happy. To be able to hold a job and live on his own. I guess those would be my goals."

Les answered, "I worry about his future. I'm always afraid that somebody will do something to him. He can't talk, and he wouldn't be able to tell us if something happened. . . ." Her lower lip quivered; she stopped. I squeezed her hand and tried to give her a peppy smile, but a block rose in my throat. We sat mutely for a good minute.

The doctor merely nodded. Sherry, eyes wet, smiled encouragingly.

Dr. Cohen said, "I suppose you know why we're here. I understand that you had a bad experience with medication in the past. But I would like you to reconsider."

Now it was our turn to be chilly. "It's a horrible thing to watch your little child going through withdrawal," I said. "We will never put him through something like that again. And frankly, we're getting really tired of doctors implying that we're doing something wrong if we don't drug him. 'We can't figure out what to do with this kid, so let's just sedate him.'"

Realizing how hostile I sounded, I backtracked a little. "I don't want to say we'll never use meds again, but only as a last resort. We should work harder to find some behavioral solution first. He's not just some lab animal."

Dr. Cohen stayed cool. "I understand why you're defensive. But you must realize that not all medications are the same. Every child responds differently to each medication. There is a new drug, Risperdal, that has shown quite dramatic results with children like Cameron. I treated one boy who had to wear pads on his arms, and so did all of his aides. He couldn't learn much of anything because his behaviors were so disruptive. We put him on Risperdal, and when I saw him again six months later, he didn't seem like the same boy. His parents said it was a miracle: he was calm, he was learning, even his speech had improved. So if we can find the right medication for Cameron, I truly believe that we can help him. I wish you would consider it."

He gave us some photocopied material on medications and a review article about new autism drugs. The research did suggest that Risperdal (risperidone) had helped aggressive kids like Cam, minus the older drugs' dangerous side effects: oversedation, tardive dyskinesia (involuntary and sometimes permanent tics, jerks, muscular movements), or neuroleptic malignant syndrome (a serious, potentially lethal acute feverish reaction).

Over the next week we reread the literature and talked at length. I kept remembering those hives, chills, and night sweats. But two arguments finally prevailed: (1) if the drug really might help Cam, we'd be negligent not to try it; (2) if we didn't try it, the school would probably kick him out. So we made up our minds to give Risperdal a shot. We really had little choice: we'd tried just about everything else.

Both of us remained uneasy about side effects, and on that first night— April 27, 1998—we carefully read the instructions on the bottle before Les measured the dose of the liquid formula. Ten minutes after she administered it, Cam's eyes grew glassy. "Bed," he said drowsily. Five minutes later, he was sound asleep.

The doctor had warned us that the drug might sedate Cam at first. But his eyes had seemed so dull and drugged that, before we headed to bed, I examined the bottle and spoon on the kitchen counter. "Hon, how much did you give him?"

"A quarter of a teaspoon, just like it says."

"It says to give him 1/4 of a milliliter. Is that the same as a quarter of a teaspoon?" I thumbed through the almanac looking for measurements. Oh no: she'd given him four times the prescribed dose!

I'd love to write that I calmly reassured my wife that it wasn't her fault, that anyone could make such a mistake the first time. But in fact I shouted at her.

"What the hell were you thinking? How could you give him four times the right dose? Jesus Christ, Les, you fucking poisoned him!" Her terrified face soon shamed me into silence.

Then we looked at each other and raced to Cam's room, certain he'd be lying there dead. But he was just snoring away. Les called the Poison Control Center and explained in a quavering voice what had happened. They checked their information—not extensive, since Risperdal was a new drug—and told us he'd probably just sleep it off. That was reassuring. They added that it might be a good idea to check on him periodically to make sure he was breathing. That was not reassuring.

During my shift, I sat tensely by my son's bed, alert for any sign that his breathing was shallow or labored. I felt his pulse—slow but strong. As I touched his warm little arm, a tide of emotions surged up inside of me: anxiety over the new drug, anger at our mistake, guilt for shouting at my wife, sorrow over my son's disorder and the agony it caused him. I flashed back to a photo we'd taken just after Cam's birth. I'm lying on my back, our tiny baby's head resting under my chin, his feet at my waist. If only I could protect him as I had then! Goose flesh rising on my arms, I gave in to racking sobs.

Wrapped in his green comforter, my son slept soundly. The next morning he was the same as ever.

The drug worked at once. Cam was calmer, easier to manage. He could concentrate and work for longer stretches. He slept better, his moods leveled out, and his aggressive episodes became shorter and less frequent. Within a week, he was named Most Improved Student.

Largely because of Risperdal, the summer of 1998 was an idyllic interlude in our life with autism. We had hired a nanny with a social work degree and wide experience to spend four hours a day playing with Cam and taking him to the swimming pool. Anita Parker was ideal: warm and friendly but firm. She was not intimidated by Cam's tantrums and praised him lavishly when he did well. Most important, he liked her.

Over the next year he continued to benefit from Risperdal. The only drawback was that it increased his appetite, so our once-slim child sported a roll of fat around his middle. With his tan and tummy, he resembled a chubby little otter.

It seemed we had jumped off the Red Queen's treadmill.

But in July 1999, Cam suddenly grew listless. He didn't want to get out of bed. He had no energy. He didn't even want to eat. Though he had no fever, no runny nose, no stomach ache, he was severely constipated. Dr. Archer, our pediatrician, prescribed Milk of Magnesia. Cam's lethargy abated.

Two weeks later it returned, worse than before. His days were little more than groggy interludes between long naps. For two straight nights, he slept for twelve hours and the next day didn't want to get out of bed at all. We hustled back to Dr. Archer. If Cam hadn't come around within two days, he said, we should consider altering the Risperdal dosage. By all means, though, he said, consult Dr. Cohen.

"I don't like the sleepiness," Dr. Cohen said. "I'm a bit concerned that it may be building up in his system. I would like you to go get liver function and blood tests immediately—today if you can—and call me back when you get the results."

All the anxiety left over from the Klonopin nightmare came flooding back. Risperdal was a new and relatively untested medication. What if we really *had* poisoned our son?

The blood tests showed nothing abnormal. Nevertheless, Cohen recommended that we take Cam off Risperdal.

Right away the banished Cam returned. That first weekend he kept his fingers jammed into his ears, as if trying to muffle disturbing sounds the drug had muted. Did he feel, as other autistic people testify, that his "brain was too loud"? Or was he just unbearably anxious?

The constantly revving engine that the drug had slowed also started up again. Cam was edgy, ready to explode at the slightest provocation. His moods careened from giddiness to rage. On Sunday he had two hour-long episodes of bouncing on the bed, then tore chunks from his mattress and cried inconsolably for fifteen-minute spells. During one crying jag, he wrenched out a large handful of Leslie's hair.

On Monday we reported our dreadful weekend to the doctors, who recommended resuming the Risperdal at a reduced dosage—less than half of what Cam had been taking. In two or three days, he had removed his fingers from his ears, but his moods remained volatile, his demeanor hyperactive.

And so, a year and a half after beginning the drug, we were back almost to where we'd started: no worse, perhaps even a little better, but even more wary of medications.

Things Go Better?

Risperdal had yielded a few more bright moments at school: one day Cam even rode the water taxi to the Inner Harbor with his classmates and was even relaxed enough to sit on Santa's lap. But overall it was more of what we'd seen at Timberland.

We knew Cam's problems weren't all their fault, knew better than anyone how "challenging," as the euphemism has it, our son could be. Even so, the staff often seemed inept or obtuse, constantly refighting old battles or failing to grasp what seemed obvious. For example, in early 1999 we met with Cam's teacher to ensure that the school curriculum matched our revived home program. No such luck: whereas at home he was given a picture and asked to match it to a word, at school he was asked to do the opposite. No wonder he was confused. He was having a lot of trouble on a matching drill. I looked at the teacher's notes: they were forcing him to do a drill he'd mastered at home two years earlier.

Leslie and I, neither of us with a special ed background, were designing the curriculum for our severely disabled son. And the staff at his Blue Ribbon school couldn't carry it out. We learned how the school really operated. The folks with the doctorates focused on administrative chores or research, while the hands-on tasks fell to young people just out of college—the only ones who'd work for their low salaries. They were ostensibly trained in behavior management techniques and had at least BAs in appropriate fields. But these raw youths were thrown into classrooms with the most difficult children imaginable. Was there really much chance they'd succeed?

A video taken at school in the spring of 1999 illustrates these problems. Cam wears a weighted denim vest that is supposed to help him sense his body and reduce his stims and aggression. The background hums with chatter, punctuated by loud squeals. Cam sits facing a ponytailed young man named Ron. This appears to be a training session for Ron.

Ron asks Cam to trace a line on an erasable slate, but the pupil is paying no attention: he seems mesmerized by something off camera. Ron nudges Cam's chin, tries to block his eyes, but Cam's head remains motionless.

The camera operator/trainer tells Ron to reward Cam with a Sweetart for paying attention. But when Ron turns his head ever-so-slightly to listen to the instruction, Cam pops the chalk into his mouth. Ron squeezes Cam's cheeks to make him spit it out, but when he again turns to listen to directions, cat-swift

Cam snatches the other piece of chalk and crams it into his mouth. When Ron finally shows Cam the Sweetart, he grabs the chalk and scribbles on the slate. But the next time Ron's attention is diverted, Cam again stuffs the chalk into his mouth. They repeat this pattern for several more trials. This is called success. Cam's reward: selecting a Language Master card for a drink of water.

Cam eventually completed his task, but responded only to tangible rewards, and even then lost focus within seconds. He used his lightning reflexes and shrewd intelligence only to disrupt and delay. Once again the million-dollar question arises: why can't or won't he use that intelligence productively? In fact, he seemed to be teasing Ron—testing him, teaching him. My son repeatedly outsmarted the teacher, who seemed to assume the boy was stupid. And this guy was going to help Cam develop his skills?

The next scene shows our son working more successfully with a female occupational therapist.

"We're going to buy a Coke," she announces, miming drinking.

Cam claps his hands, says "Aa-aah, hee," rocks sideways in his chair, plays with the rubber tube they've placed around his neck (designed to give him something to bite besides others' hands).

She helps him page through a large book of photos. At the bottom of each page is an array of coins, at the top a picture of something he can buy with them—a bag of chips, a soda.

"Where's Coke?" she asks. "We are going to buy Coke."

Cam utters his happy noises, "Uu loo loo." He's concentrating hard, but can't find it. The OT turns back to the beginning of the book; Cam growls and gnaws hard on the tubing.

They begin again, but Cam stares off. "Cameron! Where's Coke?" she asks, pointing to the picture. He looks at the book in typical fashion, his head turned to catch it at the edge of his vision. He rocks, vocalizes, bites the tubing, clears his throat loudly, claps, stares.

She tries again, "Where's Coke?" Cam looks at the page, claps. He knows darn well this is the Coke picture, but can't seem to tell his body to touch the picture. Finally he touches the bright red Coke picture. She hands him a plastic sandwich bag full of coins. If he matches the coins, he gets to buy the Coke. Cam fumbles with the bag, then lapses into the smoothing gesture he uses to strip twigs.

"Cameron, open," she says, giving the ASL sign for "open." He tries for a couple of seconds, then starts smoothing again. She opens the bag and asks him to put the coins on the table; he complies. "Good boy!" she enthuses. Cameron smiles faintly, sways in his chair—a happy gesture—and rubs his nose.

She holds up the coin in front of his face. He plugs his ears, gutturally says, "That's good, that's good," from the side of his mouth—Cameron Bogart. After

several more seconds of delaying, at last he matches the coin to the picture.
"Good!"

"Oooh, wee, looh," he replies in a throaty whisper.

One by one he matches the other coins, meanwhile clapping, rocking, plugging his ears or rubbing his nose. Finding the page with Coke and matching seven coins takes five minutes. But he *does* pay attention.

In the break room, he slips coins into the vending machine and pushes the button. At last an ice-cold can of Coca-Cola thumps down to the bottom of the bin. Cam grabs it.

Maybe the old jingle was right: maybe things *do* go better with Coke.

These would be considered good sessions. Cam is not aggressive and sporadically pays attention. But the teachers are just tools for him to obtain sweet treats, and they spend most of their time deterring him from what he really wants to do: stim, stare, clap, rock, gnaw, giggle, and chatter to himself. Anything but learn.

Is this seeming lack of motivation a cause or a consequence? Obviously, Cam's neurological problems—his executive dysfunction, weak working memory, poor fine-motor skills, sensory distortions—make comprehension and retention difficult. When you fail repeatedly, when learning demands a concentration you can barely muster, when you're distracted by lights, sounds, and smells you can't identify, you naturally resist. The remarkable thing, then, is not that he had trouble with academic skills but that he could perform any of them. Alas, the next day he was just as likely to do worse as better. Is it any wonder that much of his education degenerated into behavioral triage? Is it any wonder that the teachers got discouraged?

Yet we still felt his potential hadn't been tapped and never stopped hoping that maybe this program or that therapy would trigger a breakthrough. So we kept on running.

Have a Biscuit?

After her run with the Red Queen, Alice is very thirsty. "Have a biscuit?" says the Queen, giving Alice a hard, dry one.

"While you're refreshing yourself," said the Queen, "I'll just take the measurements." And she took a ribbon out of her pocket . . . and began measuring the ground. . . .

"At the end of two yards," she said . . . "I shall give you your directions—have another biscuit?"

"No, thank you," said Alice: "one's quite enough!"

"Thirst quenched, I hope?" said the Queen.

—*Through the Looking-Glass*

We began making regular visits to Callaway Carver Institute's outpatient psychiatric clinic, hoping that behavior therapy might eventually let us take Cam off meds.

Down the hall from the psychiatric unit was the Center for Feeding Disorders. Patients passed us on their way in or out. These kids were hard to look at. There was a grotesquely obese girl of about ten who sat glumly in a wheelchair, sometimes brushing with fat hands the wispy, light brown hair surrounding her blank moon face. There was also a tiny, shrunken boy in a motorized chair. He looked to be about four; I later learned that he was fifteen years old.

"It could be worse," I told myself.

We also encountered other psychiatric patients. One young man we never saw gave forth raspy shouts from behind a door. What was most disturbing was not the nerve-grating volume or regularity of his roars but the sound itself, a blood-chilling cross between a wildcat's snarl and a violent retch.

A nurse told me, "One day he went on like that for three hours. It just about drove everybody crazy." What agony fueled these cries? What was he trying to say?

And there was a teenaged boy sitting with his mother, a tired-looking woman with watery eyes and a half-grown-out dye job. The boy's head lolled and his tongue protruded from his mouth as he tried, with gnarled hands and vague gestures, to convey a request: "Uull, aaahh booo gaahh." His mother gave him a drink of her soda, but he continued to moan and whimper.

She spoke to him as though he were a normal preschooler. "Are you hungry? All this just because you didn't get more crackers!"

The boy began to cry.

"Oh, don't be such a bawl baby!" she scolded, hugging him with her left arm.

This boy's physical disabilities had rendered him unintelligible and, to many people, repulsive. But to his mother, he was simply her precious child. She accepted him as he was.

I admired her immensely.

I felt a pang of guilt: what was my adorable kid doing here among these desperate people with their terrible disorders? Was he lucky after all? Was he really disabled?

Then I was brought up short by the realization that we were here because Cameron was, though in a less visible way, just as impaired. He was one of them. And so was I.

During sessions, the staff put Cam in a room with a two-way mirror, and someone took data from the adjoining room. A therapist would try to engage him—ask him to play a music tape, throw a ball, or add ears to a Mr. Potato Head—or prompt aggression. Cam responded to most stimuli the same way:

by chewing on his shirt, slapping the therapist, running to the locked door and turning the handle, climbing up on the window sill to gaze out at the parking lot.

The sessions were painful, but we continued them, because the long-term plan was . . . well, that was the problem. The psychologists never explained their plan. At the initial consultation, Dr. Moran had said they'd compile data to determine what antecedents prompted Cam's aggression, find skills that might give him alternatives to "stimming" with cords or bushes, then start suitable treatments. Six months later, they were still taking data.

Leslie began to question me: what are you doing there? Why haven't they come up with something yet? She insisted on accompanying us to our next session.

In our history with professionals, I've usually played the brusque, all-business parent and Les the warm, friendly one. The good-cop/bad-cop routine had worked pretty well. This time we switched roles.

She opened decisively, "We're very concerned that these sessions have gone on for several months with nothing to show for them. We assume that you're coming up with some kind of plan or procedure. What is the overall aim?"

Dr. Moran, a tall, stressed-looking woman in her forties, glanced down at her notes. "We are trying to determine the antecedents to his aggressive outbursts. I realize it seems like all we do is take data, but experience has shown that the more data we compile, the better picture we get of the disorder and the more information we have about how best to treat it."

"That's all fine; I understand why you need the data. But enough is enough. It's time to start treating the problem instead of just recording it. We want to start seeing some results."

"But you see, the data may change from month to month; it's much more statistically sound to compare data from several time-periods. That way we can devise a treatment that accounts for most variables."

"I hate to be blunt, but this isn't cheap. We come here twice a week and each time it costs both us and the insurance company. Where's the incentive to end it?"

The doctor turned up her chin. "We are trying to help the children. We're not in it for the money."

I tried to mediate. "We know you guys are very good at what you do. But we've planted the seeds; now we think it's time for the harvest." Nobody was impressed with my metaphor.

"My husband is being nice. We are desperate. We need you to help us. Please." Whether it was Les's moist eyes or her thin-lipped assertiveness that did the trick, at the next session the doctors offered us a hypothesis.

Cam's aggression, they felt, was a product of frustration: he used it to get out of demanding situations and convey fear and anxiety. Well, we'd known that already.

We complained that the institute was too artificial, that they couldn't get an accurate picture there, so Dr. Moran agreed to start observing Cam at school and promised that by the spring of 1999 she'd have a behavioral protocol for us to follow.

The plan seemed sensible, and it gave us a reprieve from these stressful hospital visits. The next week we began to get periodic notes saying that Dr. Moran had observed Cam for forty-five minutes, or an hour and a half. After a couple of months she unveiled her protocol—da da-da dah! The basket hold. Her assistant demonstrated: take the aggressive child gently to the floor, squat behind him, hold his arms to his sides and press down so that his head is positioned between his knees. It doesn't hurt the kid (though it must feel awkward and demeaning), but keeps him from doing more damage to others or himself. You have to watch for head butts, but if it's applied correctly, they assured us, even a small woman can perform it on a fairly large child.

That was it: the result of nearly a year's therapy and observation. The vaunted Callaway Carver staff had little advice about how to prevent outbursts ("Cameron is a very anxious child with very limited leisure and imaginative skills who is subject to explosive episodes"; we'd already known that, too) and nothing to say about his long-term prognosis. But we all learned to administer the basket hold.

Cam so hated being immobilized, so hated having others' hands on him, so hated feeling helpless, that, far from calming him down, the hold made him feel bullied and abused. After two months, we gave it up.

Our Red Queens had taken ample measurements, talked authoritatively, and handed out a remedy that not only didn't allay the problem but often made it worse.

Have a biscuit.

Hold that Basket!

"But I don't want to go among mad people," Alice remarked.
"Oh, you can't help that," said the Cat: "we're all mad here. I'm mad. You're mad. . . . You must be, or you wouldn't have come here."
—*Alice in Wonderland*

As months passed, the basket hold became a symbol of the mad, mad, mad, mad autistic world we lived in, where Cam's communication disorder seemed to get transferred to everyone who worked with him.

A few months after our institute treatments had ended, we met to approve Cam's IEP and confirm his placement for the next year. The "team" included Cam's teacher, therapists, the county's special ed supervisor, and the officer who ensures that the school complies with the county's wishes.

Cam's teacher—a new woman named Shelley, hired for a program called START designed for children with serious behavior problems—gave a heartening report: Cam was controlling his outbursts better and getting along with his peers. She spoke of Cam as if were a regular kid, sprinkling her educational jargon with slang—"He's, like, really smart"—and peppering her responses with "Cool!"

Shelley found Cam to be a "promising" student, which meant that the next year, when he moved to middle school, he'd still be in an academic class, instead of being placed on a vocational track. Why wouldn't we want the school to find a noble vocation for our little novice? Because the word refers not to the discovery of some fulfilling purpose, but to programs that teach adolescents to sort laundry, wash dishes, clean floors, and put away trash—the "vocations" to which the intellectually disabled are consigned. We were relieved: our son hadn't yet been culled into the "we can't do any more for him" bin.

The compliance officer was suitably officious, but her severe demeanor softened when telling us how Cam had played with her the previous week. She'd been trying to fingerprint all students (for safety reasons); at Cam's turn, he'd put out his hand, then withdrawn it and laughed—teasing her.

"Cameron is funny. It's nice to see, since so many of the kids don't have the cognitive ability to have a sense of humor."

Our high spirits dissolved when she reached the behavioral portion of the IEP and read aloud the page-long description of the basket hold.

We politely let her finish. Then Les said, "But we have a new protocol."

"We're no longer doing the basket hold," I added.

That was the first she'd heard of it. She sent the speech pathologist to find the memo with that information, while Shelley, Leslie, and I described the new protocol, in which Cam used a "break" card. The officer apparently hadn't been listening a few minutes earlier when Shelley had outlined this technique.

We left the meeting disgruntled, but, with expectations lowered by experience, we just shrugged and vowed to maintain our home program at all costs. Later that day I got a call from a school aide, who told me that during a field trip Cam had thrown a tantrum and bitten a staff member. They'd had to perform "several basket holds" on him. It was all I could do not to scream at her, "We're not doing the basket hold any more, you nitwit!" But I only apologized and told her he was probably hot and tired and needed to pee.

Why were they were still performing the basket hold months after we'd agreed to discontinue it? Why couldn't these people talk to each other? Why couldn't they follow through on their own ideas?

The authorities' evasions, euphemisms, and empty promises—all disguising the ugly truth that they had no idea how to help our son—were just as mystifying, just as frustrating as the commands of Alice's bullying monarch. Their words may have preserved their jobs and protected their institutions, but they kept us perpetually running the Red Queen's race.

Chapter 10

Camp Wonder

All torment, trouble, wonder, and amazement
Inhabits here: some heavenly power guide us
Out of this fearful country!
—Shakespeare, *The Tempest*

The Fearful Country

One evening in early 2000 Cam burst through the door and planted himself before me.

"Dawwy hone," he declared.

"Daddy is home, Cam. I'm right here. Everything's okay. I'm just watching the news."

He changed his inflection. "Dawwy hone?"

"Cam, Daddy is already home. You're looking right at him."

I was pretending not to understand that he meant "When is Mommy coming home?" I'd been wondering the same thing, but was childishly irritated that he had mixed up "Mommy" and "Daddy," as if I wasn't getting credit for being a devoted dad. And though I knew Les had no control over the length of her work days, I was peeved at her for another late homecoming.

"Dawwy! Hone!" He was almost shouting now, his face twisted, his brown eyes blinking rapidly as he gnawed on the holder of his "suckie."

99

I squatted in front of him. "What's my name, Cam?"

"Camra," he said.

"No. *You're* Cameron. *I'm* Daddy."

"Dawwy."

"What's my name?" His mouth fell open; he was totally baffled. "I'm Daddy."

"Dawwy hone. Dawwy hone."

"Daddy *is* home," I said again.

Why didn't I take him for a ride, put on a CD, reassure him that his mom would be home soon? Maybe I wanted to punish him or punish my wife. Or perhaps I wanted to punish myself for failing to give Cam what he needed—whatever that was.

"Dawwy hone!" His lips quivering, his nose running, Cam rocked furiously in the loveseat and pounded on its arms. "Dawwy hone! Dawwy hone! Dawwy hone!" he cried, slapping his chest with each exclamation.

Suddenly my pent-up frustration at all the failed therapies, the years of feeling trapped and abandoned, boiled over. Would this kid never understand anything? I bent over and bellowed at him: "Daddy is home, goddamn it! Daddy *is* home, home, home today and every fucking day of every fucking year of this horrible fucking life!"

Cam's face crumpled and he began to blubber. He shouted one last time: "Dawwy hone!"

"Shut up! Just shut up!" I stomped into the kitchen and punched in the number of Les's cell phone.

"You get your ass home right now," I shouted. "I don't care where you are or what you are doing. You come home right NOW!" Panting, I slammed down the phone. A red cloud seemed to envelope the room.

As I gazed at Cam, rocking and slapping his chest, this portrait of innocent misery penetrated my angry haze. Instantly my rage gave way to a remorse so strong that I literally staggered. Here was my son, a ten-year-old who couldn't even call his own mother by name. And instead of responding to his need, I had mocked it.

I hung my head, then hugged my son. "Daddy's sorry, Cam. Daddy's so sorry. Mommy's on her way. She'll be home soon."

"I sowwy," he agreed—in other words, "you should be sorry."

When Les arrived home twenty minutes later, I apologized to her, too, and then we talked at length—one of many such talks over the next two years. The gist was always the same: I alleged that she gave too much to her job and not enough to us; she claimed I wouldn't let her quit work because I was too worried about money; I said I carried too much of the child-care load; she reminded me that she'd borne most of it when Cam was younger. We were both right.

Beneath the recriminations was a stark fact: we felt like prisoners, and this was our life.

Cam *had* made academic progress in the past two years. He now consistently used his Language Master to choose destinations and tasks; his receptive language had improved, and, if you gave him a limited number of concrete choices, he could answer yes/no questions. He was learning some self-help skills. He loved to swim and jump on the trampoline.

But these improvements were so gradual and so labor-intensive that they were hard to celebrate. Les had never recovered from the two years of sleepless nights that had thrown her immune system out of whack and given her constant sore throats and sinus infections. I believed I was handling things well, but I carried a massive burden of rage and sadness.

Our families tried to be supportive, but they lived thousands of miles away and were understandably frightened and confused by Cam's disorder. We joined support groups, but at those meetings every other child seemed to be doing better than ours. The meetings only deepened our guilt: if our son wasn't recovering, we must be doing something wrong. The guilt drove us to further exertions, which worsened our fatigue.

Les and I had grown estranged from each other and from the world. You can't cultivate friendships when babysitters shrink from your child and you're too exhausted go out. Isolation and rigidity, anxiety and anger: Cam's autism had spread to the entire household.

And now summer loomed—another summer when I'd be home most of the time with my son. Something had to give; we had to find respite.

A few weeks later, we attended a camp fair, where we were given brochures, videos, and other information about various summer programs. Most featured hiking, crafts, rafting, games, riding—all things that Cam couldn't or wouldn't do. What camp would tolerate his destructive behaviors, heavy stims, and explosive temper? We weren't optimistic. Yet there were two camps in Pennsylvania specializing in more "severely challenged" children. We set up appointments.

Scouting

On a Saturday in May, we drove 450 miles—into northern Pennsylvania and back. As we tooled along the Pennsylvania Turnpike, I recalled our first camp experiment, five years earlier: a day camp catering to kids with developmental disabilities. It had two swimming pools, a couple of wide playing fields, ponies, an experienced and personable staff. It was expensive—more than a thousand dollars for a few weeks—but we had hoped it would give Cam some structure and us some blessed relief. Maybe he'd even learn to play with other kids.

But after three days, the assistant director told us Cam wouldn't join any circle activities and stayed agitated most of the day, calming down only to swim or eat. He was running the staff ragged with his aggression and mood swings. Two days later, we pulled him out.

So our expectations were modest: we didn't dare hope Cam might thrive at camp, but only that he'd tolerate it. In truth, we needed it more than he did.

The first stop: Camp Quaker, two hundred miles from our home. The director—a tall, athletic blonde in her forties wearing a badge saying "Veronica Larch, MA"—showed us around. She talked nonstop, highlighting features that appealed to most parents: safety ("all our staff are trained in CPR"), education ("we'll do our best to fulfill the goals on his IEP"), structure ("his days will be fully planned"), diversity ("our staff is a mixture of American and international individuals"), diet ("one of our international staff said that in his country our dining hall would be a four-star restaurant"), and entertainment ("Paul Torney is nationally known"). At the end of the tour, she showed us a nifty promotional video packed with endorsements from parents and shots of contented campers, mostly teens and adults whose "activities" involved sitting quietly. Would our loud, hyperactive ten-year-old fit here?

The personable Ms. Larch surely believed in her camp's mission. But by this time we'd encountered enough well-meaning but unqualified people to recognize another one right away. When Cam yanked off his tennis shoes, she gaped and shook her head. A few minutes later we gave him a piece of rubber tubing to chew on.

"What's with the rubber thing?" she asked. "Why would he want to do that?"

These are mild and common behaviors for autistic children. How would she react if Cam launched into one of his bull charges?

At the top of Camp Quaker's gently sloping hill sat a roomy lodge and mess hall. At the bottom lay the eight-bunk cabins and pool. Between the mess hall and cabins was a shallow pond, which filled the air with odors of stagnant water and goose dung. There was too much open space for Cam, and the ponds looked dangerous. I imagined a posse of irate campers lined up to throttle our son after one night of his incessant clapping and peeing on everything in sight.

Cam would never be a Quaker.

A swift trip down the turnpike brought us to Camp Wonder, where a chubby young woman walked up to us and stuck out her hand. "Hi, I'm Trisha Lyndale, the director of Camp Wonder."

I winced inwardly: she looked like a college girl.

A few teenagers timidly rode herd on four younger kids while a group of disabled adults sat around in lawn chairs. It resembled a sleepy afternoon at a nursing home or one of those family reunions where the old folks repose heavily in the shade while reminiscing about the Great Depression. The staff looked totally untrained. It turned out, however, that they weren't staff but high-school kids volunteering for the day. And the disabled adults were there only for the weekend; they wouldn't be camping with our son.

In fact, the longer we looked, the better we liked Camp Wonder. Here were paved trails, an enormous new pool, and cabins housing only two campers—quite a contrast from the smelly expanses and crowded cabins at Camp Quaker.

Teddy, a chunky teen with black hair and glasses, would be Cam's counselor if he came. He knew a lot about the place: his mother was the cook, and he'd stayed here every summer for many years. And he'd already befriended Cam, who'd taken a shine to their large, chair-like swing. Teddy pushed Cam on the swing, kept track of his shoes, and shared a soda with him while Les and I finished the tour.

Camp Wonder seemed tolerant, and the staff had experience with autistic children; several kids around Cam's age had already enrolled.

On the way home, we asked Cam his opinion. "Buddy, that was camp! Did you like it?"

No answer.

"Did you like Teddy?"

"Teddy."

"Did you like him?"

"Like him." A faint smile.

Was he answering or just echoing? No matter. It was decided: he was going to Camp Wonder.

There was one scary moment that had nothing to do with the decision. Or maybe it did. As we wearily hurtled down the interstate at 70 miles per hour, near the end of this very long day, Cam began to push on Les's seat and kick her headrest. Then he turned toward me. The car veered to the left as his left foot struck my right shoulder.

"Yikes! Buddy, calm down. We're on the way home." I dodged the foot and kept driving.

Two days later I called Trisha to reserve a week's spot, starting on June 18. If the week went well, Cam would stay for a second week. If not, we were only two hours away.

Unhappy Campers

As the date for departure grew nearer, questions nagged at us. Could Cam handle overnight camp? Could the camp handle *him?* Les and I had spent exactly one night together away from him in the nearly eleven years since his birth. Would *we* be able to handle it?

A couple of events proved to us that we had to try it. The first was a meeting of a parents' group at Cam's school, designed to improve communication between us and the school staff.

Most of us were well-educated professionals. We were earnest; we were productive; we were in pain. The father of a boy in Cam's class, a lawyer named David Goodman, suggested that we take turns describing what we wanted from the group. Several parents spoke, including Rita Brooks, whose autistic teenaged son, Keith, was an "eloper"—he ran away when he got anxious. A big kid, Keith had massive shoulders developed from his habit of holding his arms over his head. His school had been unable to manage him, and Rita had been keeping him home for over a year. But now he had severe separation anxiety: if his mother even went out to the car, he'd pound on the doors and windows. One day when Rita went to fetch the mail, Keith smashed the glass on their front door.

She spoke with a resigned air, even chuckling occasionally, but her shaking voice and red face plainly attested to her suffering. We all nodded sympathetically: our details might have been different, but each of us had a similar story.

Other parents didn't need to share their stories; their appearance said everything. Martha Kaminski, the mother of a boy in Cam's class, had recently been hospitalized for exhaustion and depression. For the past two years, she'd managed her son's home program *and* helped out in his classroom. She had strived and sacrificed, yet her son was as disabled as ever. Colorless and washed out, her mouth frozen in a permanent frown, Martha gazed blankly around the room. Her husband, a tall, dark fellow with a black mustache, hunkered in the corner, his brown eyes saying, "Please don't ask me anything. I just want to be left alone."

A short while after Rita finished, a stooped man with thick half-glasses arrived, a hospital name tag with the words "Dr. Raymond Carpenter, Pathology" attached to his shirt pocket. He said hello, then mumbled something I couldn't make out. When I said, "Pardon?" he just peered at me over his glasses. He never again met my eyes.

Dr. Carpenter contributed ideas to the meeting but gazed into the corner of the room whenever he spoke. Between sentences, he *awwed* and *hmmed* into his shirt, meanwhile fiddling with the cocktail toothpicks one mother had brought—stacking them, lining them up, pulling off their plastic tips, turning them around and around.

The meeting devolved into a battle for control between him and Goodman, who kept interrupting everyone else. When Goodman volunteered to moderate future meetings, Carpenter cut him off with a loud "no!"

If we needed evidence that autism has a genetic component, we had it right in front of us: two men with the social skills of backward six-year-olds. Doubtless their sons had made them even more antisocial: who wouldn't be angry and anxious given what they had to deal with daily? They were so immured in their own misery that they couldn't hear anyone else.

Looming behind all of us were our kids—the voiceless ones. In trying to speak for them, we only exposed our own petty jealousies, obsessions and fears, our despair, our rage and indignation. Yes, our children were what we'd made them. But we'd also been remade by them: autism had torn us down and rebuilt us in its own image. It was speaking through us.

"I swear, Ray and David act as autistic as their kids," I said to Les on the drive home. "But I know how they feel: they're desperate men."

"I kept staring at poor Martha. She looked like a ghost. Wallace, please tell me I don't look that bad."

"Of course you don't, sweets."

We held hands across the front seat. We'd just seen ourselves in a mirror. Yes, we needed a break.

The gap between the end of school and the beginning of the summer term was always tense: Cam had to adjust to the looser structure, and I had to adjust to his constant presence. That year it sealed our decision to try sleepaway camp. As I sent Les off to work with a kiss on Friday, she lingered. "I just wish I didn't have to do this. I'm a nervous wreck at the end of the day," she said.

"You and me both."

Within minutes Cam had filled a cardboard box with water and poured it over the bathroom floor. I made him clean it up, putting my hand over his and wiping with a towel.

He decided to show me how unfairly he'd been treated by throwing himself back against our new couch until I shouted at him to stop. Then, as I stood at the stove frying bacon, he stormed through the house, pounding on the walls and bellowing.

"No!" I finally shouted. "You need to go to your room until you can calm down." I grabbed him by the left hand and steered him into his room. "When you get quiet, you can come out."

The bacon cooked; my rage simmered. If he stayed like this, we couldn't leave the house. Would I be trapped inside with this gremlin all day?

As Cam sat down to eat, I warned, "If you start stomping or hollering again you're going back to your room."

He growled. Translation: "Oh, yeah!? You can't make me shut up!"

"That's it!" I shouted, and heaved him up toward the kitchen door.

On the way through the doorway, we accidentally bumped a shelf and knocked down the waffle iron and a ceramic bowl, which fell to the floor with a thundering crash. We stopped and gaped at what we'd wrought.

"God damn it! Look what you did!" I roared, then hustled him back to his room and locked the door.

Cam shrieked, kicked his walls, and beat on the floor while I graduated from red-hot rage to tight-lipped fuming. For some stupid reason, I entered his room. "Listen to me!" I said, clasping his arms. "If you don't stop that screaming you're going to stay in this room all day!" I shook his arms back and forth a half-dozen times. Then I slammed the door and paced around the house, swearing. Another jail term with an indefinite sentence.

Five minutes later, I went to let him out. That's when I noticed the scrape mark on his side where he'd bumped the shelf. And that's when I spotted the marks on his arms and tiny bruises on his chest.

"Oh my God." My heart dropped like the ceramic bowl. All the blood in my body rushed into my ears and cheeks. What had I done?

I sat on the bed, holding my son and stroking his shoulders. "Daddy's sorry," I said, rocking him in my arms. "I'm sorry, Cam." I couldn't get my breath. I hand-brushed his hair, then tentatively examined his body again. Yes, those little red spots were definitely bruises; yes, that was a scrape on his side.

For the rest of the day, I reexamined Cam every ten minutes. I could think of nothing else. The marks pulsed out their message: piss-poor father, piece of shit. I'd bruised my own son! He couldn't help himself, but what was my excuse? I spent half the afternoon sitting on the couch with my chin in my hands. How had things degenerated so far?

I called Les and told her we'd broken the bowl. Then I took a deep breath and added, "And I think I bruised Cam by gripping his arms too hard."

"What kind of bruises?"

"You know, little red squeeze marks."

"Oh God. I was worried about just this kind of thing."

"I was awful. I really lost my temper. I feel like a total jerk." I paused. "I don't know what's wrong with me."

"Autism, that's what's wrong. If anybody saw what we lived with, they'd be shocked that we've even survived. Most people would have folded long ago."

"What makes you think I'm not folding?"

I felt oddly disappointed: I wanted her to shout at me, criticize my poor judgment. Couldn't she see that I deserved to be punished? Why wouldn't she let me be a villain?

Cam forgave me too. Less than an hour after the incident, he sat beside me and put his cheek next to mine—his way of giving a kiss. But *I* didn't forgive me. The incriminating evidence glowing redly on Cam's arms proved that, for a few minutes, I'd hated my own son.

The rest of the day went smoothly: Cam was unusually calm and compliant during visits to my office, the grocery store, and gymnastics. But I was still shaken. If I have another day like this one, I told Les that night, just commit me to the mental hospital.

Wonder and Amazement

On departure day, Cam woke up at 4 a.m. and crawled into bed with us. At

8 I awoke and gazed at him sleeping beside me, marveling at his long eyelashes and sleek skin. How could I ever be angry at this angel?

Later, Les brought out Cam's new green sleeping bag. "Oohh, loo, loo," he said, crawling in head first. Then he spread it out on the floor and watched TV while lying in it. At 11:30 he went outside and sat in the car.

The hum of our anxiety grew louder. Would he get homesick? What if he gets bitten by an insect? What if he injures someone else? And what if something awful happens to him? He couldn't even tell us. We'll never forgive ourselves if we put him in danger. And then came another feeling, the guilty secret we didn't dare admit—that we'd feel liberated—and its corollary—the fear that he might enjoy camp more than home.

Which was worse? That he would miss us? Or that he wouldn't miss us?

I told friends that we expected a call on Tuesday or Wednesday: "Cam bit two counselors and a camper. We're sending him home." Or "Cam was bucked off a horse and broke his leg." Or the one I don't even want to write: "Cam was taken to the emergency room for. . . ." My mind reeled off a dozen dreadful, unlikely possibilities.

Best-case scenario: he loved it and wanted to stay another week. The odds of that happening, we felt, were about as high as those of being struck by lightning. Nevertheless, we paid in advance for two weeks. Call it blind faith.

On June 18, 2000, we sped toward Camp Wonder. Cam happily sang his repertoire.

Upon arrival, we unloaded his stuff while he made a beeline for the swing set. It was a warm, humid day, so the dining hall, crammed with campers, parents, and counselors, was stuffy. Most of the counselors looked like college kids; most campers seemed older than Cam. The whole gamut of disabilities was on display: boys and girls in wheelchairs; teens with Down syndrome; tiny men and microcephalic women with huge, puppy-dog eyes.

A short young man sat at the nurse's table and greeted us. "What's your name?" he asked thickly as he shook our hands. He wouldn't let go of Les's hand, and she stood awkwardly for several minutes while he stared at her. A heavyset woman in her fifties pulled out a bag of various pills, all labeled and slotted. Her pharmacopia made our little bottle of Risperdal look pitiful.

"Have you been here before?" she asked Leslie.

"Our son has never been away from home before," Les answered.

"He'll love it. We've been coming here for twelve years and it's just great. You two will really enjoy yourselves." Les looked ready to cry.

"Oh, he'll adjust," the lady assured us. "Now, honey, don't you sit by the phone all day," she admonished as she departed.

We went outside with Cam's stuff: a huge bag filled with clothes and toiletries, another bag of food, and two sleeping bags. I had ridiculed these preparations as overkill, but every camper seemed to have just as much.

As we brought Cam into the dining hall, his right hand shook in my grasp. We told him he'd have lots of fun and that Mommy and Daddy would be back in a week to pick him up. Then we turned him over to Teddy and walked to the car. I forced myself not to look back.

Les teared up. "I'm terrified. What if something happens to him?"

"Hon, he's going to be fine. It's the right thing to do." I recalled my excitement on the day, almost twenty years earlier, when we'd loaded up our little car and started the long trek from Montana to Atlanta. I recalled our blissful anticipation during the months of Les's pregnancy. It seemed that another new world might be opening up for us on this day. I felt exhilarated.

As we pulled back onto the interstate, a colossal thunderstorm struck. The rain strafed us relentlessly, pummeling the car with violent sheets of water. The lightning threw jagged blows down to the cowering earth. It felt like an omen. The heavens seemed to shout, "How dare you abandon your son!"

I tried to dismiss these feelings but couldn't help thinking the storm embodied our emotions: elation that we'd actually done it, terror that we were making a horrible mistake. As we neared Villanova, I tried to pass a motor home and was blinded by the jets of water it threw back. I hit the brakes and dodged back into the right lane, my hands clammy with sweat. The rain seemed to taunt us: "See what happens when you get off the treadmill?"

As the storm stayed over us most of the way home, I recalled a figure from the Sunday comics of my childhood: Joe Bftsplk, the jinx from "Li'l Abner," followed by a dark cloud wherever he went.

Unbelievably, as we neared our exit, a rainbow appeared in the sky. I knew it was merely a meteorological phenomenon, not some promise of a new covenant or an arrow pointing to a crock of gold. Yet I couldn't help but feel the heavens portended good fortune.

Then I remembered it was Father's Day.

Reflecting

Feed yourself with questioning,
That reason wonder may diminish.
—Shakespeare, *As You Like It*

Here's what I wrote in my journal on the second day of camp, June 20, 2000:

The house feels eerie: Cam's stuff is all around, but the actual boy has vanished. We're still locking all the doors, as if he's ready to burst through them any second.

Last night we dined out and had a drink, something we haven't done in more than a year. As we walked from the restaurant, I looked at my watch and asked what time it was. Then we realized that we could come home anytime we damn well pleased! It was liberating but also sobering. Who are we, anyway?

As we sat in the dark bar, Les looked up at me and said, half-smiling, "I think I've had an epiphany. Our lives are sterile and empty without Cam." She used these particular words because several years ago friends told us that after their son was born they realized that their childless lives had been "sterile and empty." We'd scoffed then, and even now I don't really believe our lives would be sterile and empty without Cam. But our house does seem tomblike and void. Apparently I now need my autistic son to define myself.

Even so, many times in the last ten years I've heartily wished we didn't have a child. Occasionally I've even asked myself, "What if somebody gave you the choice: you can go back ten years and decide not to have Cam?" Would we do it again, knowing about Cam's autism and all the pain, disappointment, frustration, sorrow, and rage that would ensue? On better days, I answer, why, sure! No matter what, he's my boy! I would never want him not to exist! On other days, I wonder if even Cam would choose to live through all this again.

When you read recovery stories or uplifting autobiographies of high-functioning autistic people, you feel that if you were truly a good parent, you'd have "beaten" autism too. But what if you don't beat it? Then what?

You can point fingers. We often did—mostly at ourselves. During one period, Les convinced herself that a kitchen solvent she'd once used had caused Cam's autism. She obsessed over it for months.

I tried to reason with her: "Hon, he wasn't even in the house that day. And you used such a minute amount. It just doesn't add up."

"But right after that is when he started to show symptoms. I just know it was that 'Goof-off' stuff. Why oh why did I use that shit?" We eventually remembered that Cam's symptoms had appeared before she'd used the solvent.

Other times she attributed Cam's disorder to her illness during pregnancy. Again she tortured herself with what-ifs: "Why did I make that trip when I was pregnant? I should have been more careful!" But there's no evidence that any prenatal illness had anything to do with Cam's disorder.

Yet it's impossible not to ask why. There are so many possibilities. Recently a number of parents and a few researchers have tried to link autism to thimerosal, a mercury compound used to preserve childhood vaccines. Mercury poisoning causes neurological problems somewhat similar to those in autism, so this explanation seems plausible. Cam cried long and hard after his first vaccination, but we don't recall any behavioral changes after any shot.

We've also wondered if some environmental toxin did it. During Les's pregnancy, we rented our house from a tobacco farmer. Was Cam's development warped by some pesticide our landlord carried on his clothes? Our hometown in Montana is now a Superfund site, having been riddled for decades by deadly asbestos dust from a vermiculite mine. One of the boys who grew up next door to me also has an autistic son. Is this a coincidence or a consequence of toxic chemicals?

It's tempting to blame nasty corporations and their toxic leaks. But it's likely that autism is at least partly genetic. Scientists are discovering abnormalities on several chromosomes associated with the kinds of deficits and distortions seen in autism. Perhaps these glitches cause the disorder, or perhaps they foster an inability to metabolize certain chemicals that eventually leads to autism. It's also probable that autism is not one disorder but many, each produced by a distinct combination of genetics and environment. If so, there's nothing anyone could have done to prevent it. Yet that's precisely why such explanations are unsatisfying.

No matter how rational you think you are, when something like autism strikes your family, you look for magical explanations. So I sometimes think, language always came easily for Les and me, so maybe God is evening things out. I once mocked a mentally disabled boy who lived in my neighborhood: am I being punished for my insensitivity?

Such explanations are more compelling because autism is so nebulous: no tumor invades your child's body, no visible deformity mars his looks. Blaming yourself gives you an illusion of control: if only *I* had done more, my child wouldn't be autistic. What a perverse sense of power guilt gives you! On the other hand, if you *can't* blame somebody or something—if you're consumed by anguish and rage without a villain in sight—you feel like a character in a Thomas Hardy novel: a helpless puppet flung around willy-nilly by a malignant or indifferent cosmos. It's much more satisfying to find a scapegoat, even if it's yourself.

So we understand why parents wear themselves out on blame crusades, empty their bank accounts pursuing fad therapies, and drive themselves to emotional breakdowns: they're trying to save their children, or at least striving to stave off their own guilt for *not* saving them.

It's only human to ask, "Why us? What did we do to deserve this?" In the early years, I did my share of cursing fate. But blame is a narcotic: at first it makes you feel better, but then it slowly devours you. Gradually we have come to grips with the most difficult recognition of all: nobody is to blame.

What else can you do? You can accept your child as he is. I'm not quite there. Even now I have fantasies of an alternate world where Cam is a typical boy. And I still resent other people's attempts to show me the silver lining, those well-meaning acquaintances who say, "He's lucky to have such good parents." Or worse: "God chose him for you." I know they're only trying to help, but I want to grab them by the shoulders and shake them. What kind of God would give a child a lifelong disability just to teach his parents a lesson? Even the world's biggest narcissist couldn't believe such a thing. Yes, Cam's disability has forced me to rethink my views about intelligence. But surely I could have learned this some other way.

Certain advocates try to convince us that autism is not a disability, but merely a different way of being human, no better or worse than any other. It's good that people on the higher end of the autism spectrum are trying to rid autism of its stigma and celebrating their uniqueness. But my son is not like them, and our world is not theirs. If I were Aladdin and had three wishes, the first would be a no-brainer: "Please, genie, take away Cam's autism and make him a regular boy!"

While Cam was at camp, Les and I slipped back into the easy intimacy of our BC (Before Cam) years: eat an informal dinner, then sit side by side on the couch reading or watching a dumb TV show. She slept through the nights, and I no longer paced nervously every evening at 6 p.m. For the first time in months, we bantered as in old times. But several times a day I eyed the phone, fighting an overpowering urge to call Camp Wonder. On June 26 I finally gave in. My journal reads,

Wonder of wonders: he's doing well! Teddy said Cam is swimming three hours a day and even riding the horses "like a pro!" I wish I were there to see it: I'm so proud of him. We've decided to let him stay for the second week. This is beyond our wildest fantasies!

It's an enormous relief not to have to be on guard every moment. Like a kid whose parents are gone for the day, I've relished doing forbidden things: leaving doors ajar, playing the saxophone in the living room instead of downstairs, not bothering to put away the shampoo, detergent, or salt (three items Cam unfailingly dumps out). Yet I know this experience is meaningful only because it's a break from routine. Eventually I'll need my parent—or in this case, my child—to return.

But here is the biggest shock of all: I miss him terribly. For several minutes today, I sat on the couch yearning for my son like an exile longing for his homeland. I miss the smell of his hair—shampoo blended with sun. I miss the feel of his long-fingered hands clasping mine. I miss his voice—the flutelike, almost sotto voce way he sings and the full-throated roar when he's in a good mood. I miss those "oooh, loohs," and those goofy laughing spells. I even miss the springing of the trampoline.

I've often felt that Cam's disability makes our lives hell. Now I'm not sure. Maybe there's something worse than having Cam around: *not* having him around.

No Place Like Home?

As we drove to camp the next Sunday, my stomach danced like a teenager's on his first date. Would Cam remember us? Would he be mad? If he was sorry to come home, we'd feel inadequate; if he was happy, we'd feel guilty. Which would be better?

At Camp Wonder our son approached us, fingers jammed into his ears. Les approached him. "Cam, honey, it's Mommy."

"Hi, buddy," I said, from a few feet away.

He glanced our way and walked right past, making for the swing set. It was hard not to feel a little rejected. Apparently, he not only didn't miss us, but even viewed us as obstacles. We put his gear into the trunk anyway. I'm not sure he knew what was happening. Maybe he thought camp had been punishment. Or maybe he thought going home was punishment. In any case, it was rewarding to hear Teddy say, "I'm requesting Cam again for next year."

"We'll definitely be back," I said.

The camper sported a dark tan, a dry scalp, and a couple of nasty-looking bug bites. Otherwise he seemed fine, and as we motored back toward Philadelphia he entertained us with a medley of his greatest hits: "No more monkeys jumping on the bed," he shouted, then launched into "Ain't gonna rain no mo'!" Halfway through, he stopped and looked at us expectantly.

"How in the heck can I wash my neck / If it ain't gonna rain no more?"

"Ha, ha, ha!"

Les and I exchanged smiles. We had our boy back.

By the time we crossed the Maryland line, however, our boy was rocking, growling, and kicking Leslie's seat.

"We're going home, hon," Les said. "We'll be there in just a few minutes, so hang on."

"Umer ohnu gim home," replied Cam. Did he want to go home or did he not want to go home? Maybe the latter: for the first few hours he was ill at ease. But pretty soon he sat down to watch a video. "Oh, yeah," his face said, "I forgot about Raffi. I really like him."

His homecoming returned us swiftly to our "normal" lives: hypervigilant attention to Cameron's every need and mood. Les and I had passed the two weeks without a harsh word. By that evening, we were bickering. I accused her of interfering when I'd asked Cam about camp. She told me I was pressuring him. Like a mooning lover, I'd felt rejected by my son, who'd wanted to hold Mommy's hand, cuddle with her, and luxuriate in the bathtub with her safely nearby. I'd foolishly expected him to show some sign of having missed me.

The next day Cam devoured an entire loaf of bread, two bowls of oatmeal, an orange, six pieces of bacon, two bowls of rice, a large Coke, a sixteen-ounce bottle of water, and half a bag of M&Ms—all *before* lunch. He also gleefully flooded the bathroom and performed his usual shenanigans in Target, burping loudly, squealing freely, and laughing impertinently. At the moment these behaviors didn't seem so bad.

The next day was July 4—Cam's eleventh birthday, the night we tried to get him to watch *The Wizard of Oz*. I couldn't help but feel he understood that the story resembled his recent experiences. "There's no place like home," Dorothy chants, then wakes up in her own bed. Cam had also returned to *his* drab Kansas. But did it feel like home? Or was it just another Oz?

A couple of weeks later Cam threw a tantrum and whacked himself repeatedly on the chest and shoulders. The next day I spotted bruises on his upper arms. Relief washed over me: these were the same kind of bruises he'd shown after our big confrontation, when I'd spent the whole day feeling guilty and ashamed.

Those bruises had been self-inflicted. A heavy load lifted from my back. I was not guilty, ladies and gentlemen of the jury!

Cam's two weeks at camp had let me reflect on my own "autism"—my obsessions, compulsions, weaknesses, disabilities. But what mattered most was not the time we spent away from him; it was the decision to send him. Sure, we'd needed a break. But the real lesson was about trust, acceptance, and, finally, love. All of Cam's life either his parents or people we supervised had been telling him what to do. In handing the reins to others, we had to trust them; and we had to trust ourselves—believe we weren't endangering our only child. Above all, we had to trust Cam, have faith in his capacity to take a leap into the unknown. We had to believe that he could, in some limited way, take care of himself.

We'd begun to realize that we couldn't cure Cam. But in abandoning that dream, we entered an even more difficult stage of our life with autism: the stage of accepting him, not as a symbol of our aspirations or a problem to be solved but as simply *himself*. In letting go, even for two weeks, we'd learned that if he was to enter the world, he'd have to do it on his own terms.

But the most surprising thing about the experience was this: Cam's sojourn in Wonderland had reawakened my love for him.

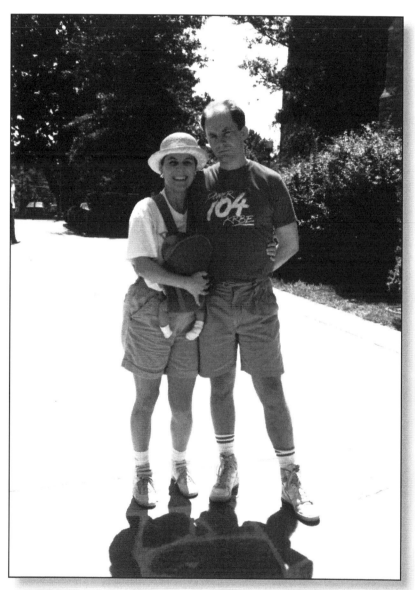

Three of us, '89

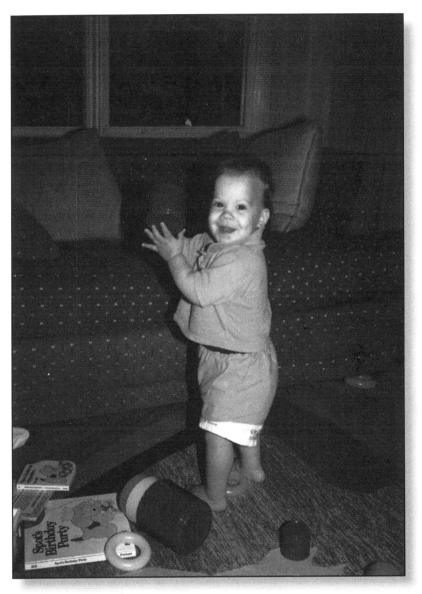

Cam at 1 in our new house

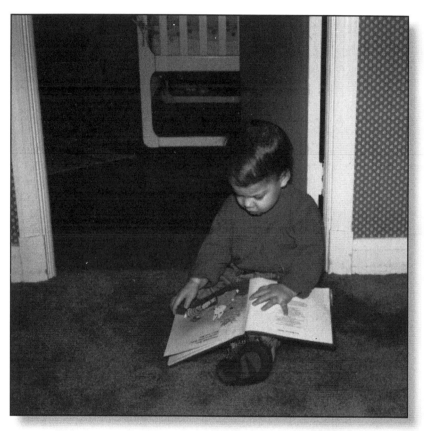

Cam's Book Club

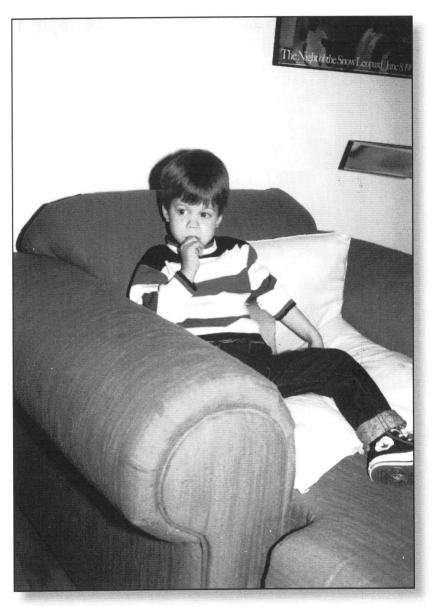

Pensive Cam at 4 ½

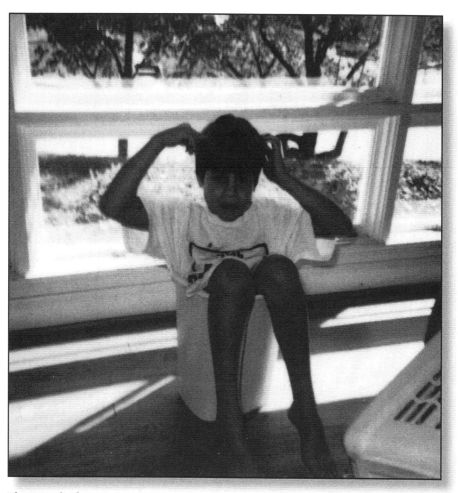

The Wastebasket Era

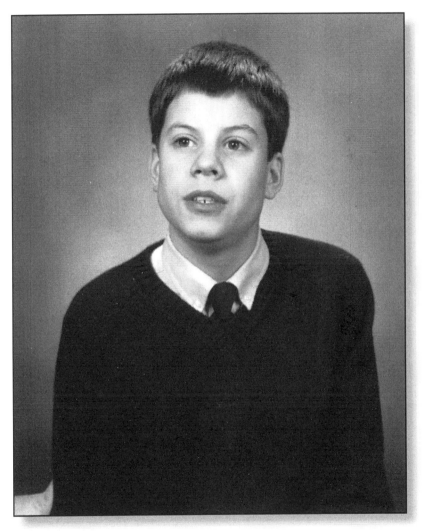

Big boy at 12

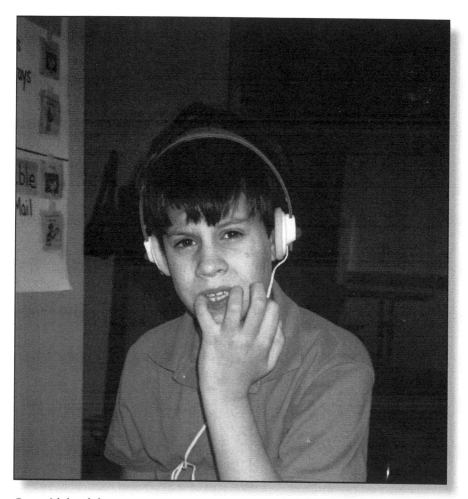

Cam with headphones

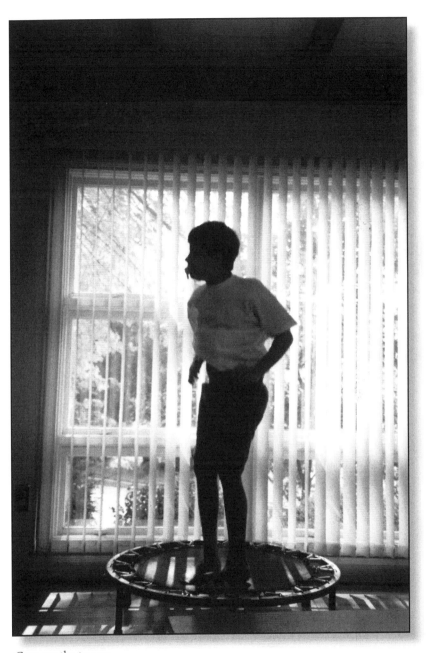

Cam on the tramp

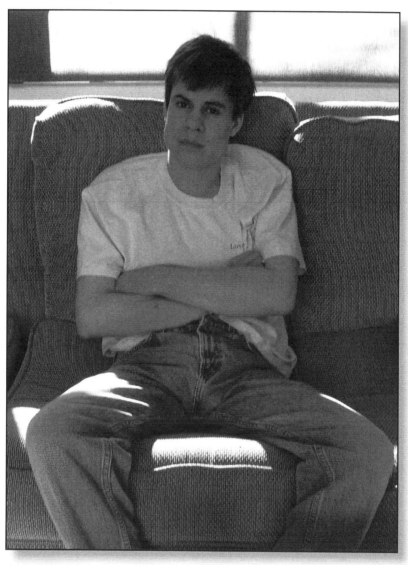

Cam at 19

Part Two

Refractions

Chapter 11

Urinetown

Only the young are allowed to suffer
openly. Adults go to a punishment room

with water but nothing to eat.
They lock the door and suffer the noises

alone. No one is exempt
and everyone's pain has a different smell.
—Craig Raine, "A Martian Sends a Postcard Home"

Not long after we learned that Cameron had autism, Leslie attended a work-shop led by a psychologist who called himself "Mr. Potty." The man boasted that he could toilet-train a kid in one day. He'd taken his methods from a book by Nathan Azrin and Richard Foxx, who recommend giving a child copious quantities of liquids and confining him or her to the bathroom. When the child seems ready to urinate, you place him or her on the toilet. With nowhere else to go, the kid quickly learns where to deposit the waste. We were confident we wouldn't need to resort to such harsh tactics. We'd take Cam's cues, and when the time was right, gently teach him to urinate and defecate in the toilet.

At the workshop Les also heard disturbing toilet-training tales from other parents:

"My son would always go in the toilet, and then suddenly he started spraying it everywhere. He was trained, then he wasn't trained."

"My son smears his feces. If he wakes up early and we don't catch him in time, he spreads poop all over his bedroom walls."

"My daughter still wears diapers at age eight. I'm desperate for a solution."

These horror stories frightened my wife, but I assumed these parents had done something wrong or that their children were more impaired than our son. I've been amply repaid for my smugness.

Basic Training

We trained Cam for bowel movements at age five, and he hasn't had an accident since. Urination was another story—a long and painful one.

When we were first training him at age four, he'd sometimes give signs that he had to pee, but other times would simply stand on the rug, gaze curiously at his penis, and let it flow. He liked to watch the water but didn't seem fully to grasp—as it were—that it was coming from him. We began to worry: he was supposed to start preschool in the fall, and the school stipulated that every child be toilet-trained. It was now or never.

I obtained Azrin and Foxx's book *Toilet Training in Less Than a Day.* After our months of struggle, their procedures no longer seemed cruel. In fact, they're designed for children who need constant repetition to get the picture, so they were tailor-made for Cam. We subjected him to the method for most of one Saturday.

As the long day passed, I recalled Craig Raine's Martian poem, and wondered if Cam shared the alien's views on toilet habits. In any case, he learned how to "suffer the noises" pretty quickly: before the day was over, he was voluntarily peeing in the toilet. Over the summer, his understanding of the process got better and better, and by fall, we had a toilet-trained kid. Even at night he'd dutifully arise from bed and pad into the bathroom. He was still inconsistent but usually peed somewhere near the toilet.

Ah, there was the rub: he didn't always go in the toilet. In fact, he seemed to delight in peeing everywhere *but* there. He'd let fly toward the corner between the bathtub and toilet or hose down the toilet seat. His favorite ploy was to aim directly at the raised seat and then stare in furrowed-browed fascination as the urine trickled slowly into the water. Of course, not all of it made its way into the toilet, and what didn't left a yellow trail and pungent scent.

When nobody was watching, he'd sneak into the bathroom and spray wherever he felt like spraying. It was as if his penis was a new toy he'd found—and look, the water goes wherever you point! I figured that as long as he urinated somewhere in the bathroom, we should be satisfied; he'd get the aim thing down eventually. I also remembered as a small boy being so thrilled by my ability to control the pressure and direction of the flow that I'd sometimes forget to aim. Anyway, what male doesn't urinate on the floor occasionally?

Going to Battle

As the months passed, the ubiquitous odor of urine began to get under Les's skin, and she started scolding Cam whenever she caught him missing the toilet. Things were degenerating in so many other aspects of our life that we vowed to hold the line on this one: "He *will* pee in the toilet. For God's sake, we've got to have some semblance of civilization around here." Eventually urination came to represent autism's control over our lives: it epitomized our failure to *make* Cam get better.

And so the bathroom became a battlefield, with Cam determined to make water wherever he wanted to make water and the two of us equally determined that he put it in the toilet instead of on the floor, in the bathtub, or behind the commode.

If we asked him to sit to urinate, he'd refuse to go, so we began following him to the bathroom, reminding him, "Put the pee in the potty, bud." Even so, he'd first irrigate the back of the toilet before tilting down toward the basin. Sometimes he'd stand on the bathtub and aim from there. Once I caught him happily firing a high arc toward the sink.

With shame, I recall another time when I grabbed him by the shoulders after he'd repeatedly urinated all over the floor. "God damn it! That's the third time you've done that today!" I yelled. "Put it in the potty!" The quivering child fled the bathroom, and for the rest of the day peed *only* on the floor.

The tougher we got, the more erratic he became. We didn't understand that once a behavior gets entrenched, it demands such enormous effort to dislodge it that you're better off ignoring it and letting it pass on its own. Nor did we understand that even the most stubborn neuro-typical people (I count myself in this group) are not in the same class as a person with autism. When it comes to fixations, Cam—like many other autistic people—doesn't respond to logic; or rather, he responds only to a private logic of strict rules and compelling obsessions.

"Where does the pee go?" we'd ask, coaxingly, pleadingly, angrily, repeatedly. "In the potty," he'd answer. But though Cam could *say* it until he was red-faced and bawling, he wouldn't or couldn't consistently *do* it.

No doubt he was confused: first we told him to go to the bathroom and then we got all worked up about it. "If I'm supposed to go in here, how come they start yelling whenever I do?"

The bathroom truly had become a punishment room.

During these first Urine Wars, my son learned a lesson he never forgot: he could make us instantly angry or happy simply by withholding or giving up his urine. We were so immersed (almost literally) in the problem that we couldn't see the connection between our heightened vigilance and his defiance—that the more attention we paid to it, the more he exploited it.

By early 1996, he commenced every Lovaas session by announcing, "Potty!" and used the same request to avoid any other unwanted task. The shrewd little dude had figured this much out: that word gets you a few minutes off. We felt we should honor his requests because it had been so difficult getting him to make them. We instructed the therapists to take him to the bathroom after the first request, but ignore subsequent ones. The result: Cam wet his pants frequently, even when he'd apparently emptied his bladder only ten minutes earlier. He'd figured out how to save some for the proverbial rainy day. Once he learned that, we were at his mercy.

It was as if all of his dammed-up play instincts had been rechanneled to his urinary tract. When he was four, we installed a large plastic climber in his room. Cam preferred not to explore it but instead found a secure perch and urinated onto the rug: our own little gargoyle fountain. We dutifully cleaned up each time, but eventually the smell became so powerful that we had to discard the rug, thereby uncovering a large patch of permanently discolored floorboards.

Cam loved carpet. Often he'd enter the living room with the sole purpose of urinating on the rug. Why rugs? Maybe because the liquid makes no sound and then vanishes. "Look! It comes out of here and then it goes there but then it just goes away. Cool!" Or maybe he agreed with the autistic author Donna Williams, who enjoyed urinating on carpet because "the more I covered the carpet, the more of a 'me' in the world there was. . . . The smell belonged to me and closed out other things." A vinegar/water mixture will dry the stain and mask the smell, but the odor of that much urine never fades entirely.

Our living room couch was another favorite target. For a long time, we doggedly tried to scour away every stain, but eventually the sheer volume of liquid overwhelmed our puny efforts. Our off-white couch became pintoed with pee stains.

We tried everything. On weekends we put him on a twenty-minute schedule, setting an egg timer that chimed when the interval ran out. Then we'd say, "Cam, do you need to go potty?" Usually he'd decline, but we'd make him go into the bathroom anyway, hoping to keep his bladder empty. Other times we ignored his urinating, reasoning that he was doing it only to get our attention. If we stopped noticing it, maybe he'd stop doing it. But after three days, we had to give up this tactic or face death by inundation.

Our ears became minutely attuned to a myriad of liquid sounds: the melodious splash of water in the toilet; the soft, spattering drizzle when urine hits the floorboards; the squish of feet on a soaked rug; the "eek" heard after sitting on a damp sofa patch.

Of course, the bathroom reeked (because urine had seeped into the floorboards and the tiny cracks around the bathtub); even worse, the smell of Cam's "pain" was so pervasive that you could detect it the moment you entered our house.

So it was that we came to live in the village called Urinetown. Mayor Cameron had ringed the village with an ammoniac aroma every bit as effective as a moat. This barrier kept all but the most intrepid visitors far away.

Urinetown was a confining place for all residents. Not only couldn't we invite guests to our place (who can enjoy a meal when enveloped by the stench of urine?), but for years one of us had to be in the room with Cam at all times so he wouldn't urinate on the furniture. If some Sunday we slipped into the den to watch *The Simpsons,* our half-hour of amusement was commemorated by an unholy trinity of new wet spots on the floor, rug, and sofa—the penalty for having fun.

Car rides have always been one of Cam's favorite activities. He sips his Coke, crunches ice, sways to music, and vocalizes his comfort sounds—"ooh wee looee, awee"—as if watching a private movie through the window. He's master of the world, safe in a climate-controlled bubble. You'd think, then, that he'd be placid and pee-free on rides. You'd be wrong.

Motor vehicles were mobile toilets. Starting at age eight, he peed in his pants on any ride longer than fifteen minutes. Perhaps he figured that if he told us he had to go potty, we'd rush home and ruin his fun. So he usually stayed mum and let it flow into his pants and onto the seat. We learned to prepare for such incidents by placing a thick towel beneath him, but some urine inevitably oozed into the upholstery. Sam the Corolla now permanently wore Cam's smudge and shared Cam's smell—the same pungent tang that perfumed our home.

Urinetown had colonized the world beyond our walls. It was becoming Urine Nation.

We had to do something. So in December 1997 we visited the Behavioral Clinic at Callaway Carver Institute, where we were assigned a doctoral student named Lisa Finch. A slender woman with jet black hair and a sharp gaze, Lisa listened attentively to our tales of woe, then crisply assured us that she could help, though she warned that the therapy would require lots of work and persistence.

She asked if Cam still wore diapers at night.

"Yeah, he wears pull-ups. We got so tired of getting up in the middle of the night to change the bed that we put them back on him a few months ago."

"I understand. But the pull-ups could be confusing him. He might not understand that it isn't okay to urinate in the bed."

Leslie and I exchanged uneasy glances. We dreaded what was coming next.

"I recommend that you throw away the diapers."

"Oh, God! We put him back in them because we were getting no sleep at all!"

"That must have been tough," replied Lisa. "But he's got to learn that the only place you urinate is in the toilet, whether you're in bed or walking around."

We'd been asking Cam sit while urinating. Lisa advised against it. "Along with the confusion there might be a sensory problem—he isn't sure when he needs to go. Getting him to stand up will help jolt him out of the pattern, and it might reassure him to actually see the urine flowing into the water."

That made sense, and the final portion of the remedy seemed equally sensible: record each time he urinated—both appropriately and inappropriately—noting antecedents and consequences. That way we could discover if he was having more "accidents" at certain times of day or at stressful moments and determine if our responses were helping or hindering.

The first consequence of these measures was, of course, nightly bedwetting. To our surprise, however, he now slept through the deluge. The data also showed that his urination increased after meals and during high-demand periods. Lisa recommended that we put him back on a twenty-minute schedule.

Over the next three months, the problem gradually improved. Standing up to urinate did seem to assure Cam that his body was working fine and that he'd actually done the deed. Taking off the pull-ups did clarify the rules. This is not to say that the problem dried up.

For example, around this time they tried a new protocol at school to combat Cam's aggression: whenever he had a tantrum he was sent to a "time-out" room to calm himself before returning to the group. But Cam enjoyed the punishment room. As soon as the door closed, he'd strip off his clothes and happily urinate on the floor: "Whee! I'm free to pee!" They abandoned this plan after two days.

By February 1998 he was down to a ten-minute reminder interval, which meant that he was almost constantly being prodded to go potty. His bathroom schedule controlled our lives. Les or I would set the timer and sit down just long enough to skim a magazine article or watch a segment of a TV show. It was like living in one of those psych experiments in which researchers ring a bell every few minutes. Your day is parceled into short waiting periods punctuated by ugly confrontations. The hours crawl by.

At the signal, she'd fetch Cam from his room or stand by the couch and hold his hand. "Okay, buddy, the timer went off, time to go potty."

Cam fought the schedule tenaciously. He'd refuse to urinate in the bathroom, then let fly on the floor as soon as he left. Or he wouldn't get off the couch, which meant we had to carry him, wailing and writhing, into the bathroom. He put five new stains on the sofa in two days. We were in despair: the new protocols were making things worse. What should we do?

Just as the rope of our nerves was ready to snap, Cam apparently decided that this surveillance took all the fun out of it. The next weekend we had nary an accident, though he stayed on the timer. Hope rose like a tattered flag. Had we finally won the potty wars?

Liquid Language

I wish I could say we had. In fact we lived in Urinetown for several more years, though the battles evolved from a blitzkrieg to frequent guerrilla skirmishes and sniper attacks. Our tactics? One: take him to the bathroom first on every outing and thereby stave off most accidents. Two: maintain hawk-eyed vigilance at home, preventing further furniture blemishes. These measures confined Urinetown to a few toxic sites.

Motor vehicles were one of them: Cam still thought of cars and buses as large, comfortable Porta-potties. During 1998 and 1999 he arrived at school most days with wet pants. Then he reversed it: for the next few years he wet his pants on virtually every ride home.

He also wet his pants on even the shortest car trips. The little internal timer that we had, with such effort, taught him to notice, went off-line as soon as he entered a car. But he didn't seem to mind and seldom made a peep before or after he peed. Short of banning rides—one of Cam's few pleasures—we saw little recourse but to ignore the wetting and quietly clean up.

Nor did the bed-wetting go away: with occasional exceptions, he wet the bed *every* night for four more years. Believe me, we did everything we could think of. We tried keeping Cam up as late as possible, cutting out fluids after 7 p.m., making him visit the toilet frequently before bedtime. Mostly these tactics just made him testy. Theorizing that a sensory issue was involved, we tried various combinations of sheets, blankets, and comforters. These experiments ended when he started shredding his bedclothes—first sheets, then blankets, and finally the plastic mattress cover. Cam had an uncanny knack for divining the one spot where the mattress was exposed. The result: a permanently smelly bed. But it seemed foolish to spend money on a new mattress as long as the bed-wetting continued. What remained of viable bed clothes were five comforters too thick for him to rip. Daily laundering soon wore out our washer and dryer.

We discovered that he usually wet the bed just as he fell asleep: it was too much trouble to rise from the warm bed and walk to the "punishment room." As soon as he peed, he'd bounce out of bed with a clap that meant "Yay for me," or "Yoohoo, I did it again," or maybe "Dang it, I really meant to get up this time."

No doubt he liked the feeling of urine oozing into the bedclothes. I ruefully recalled the beginning of James Joyce's *A Portrait of the Artist as a Young Man*, in which young Stephen Dedalus reminds himself, "When you wet the bed, first it is warm then it gets cold." Like Stephen, Cam luxuriated in the liquid warmth, and the clamminess that ensued didn't outweigh the initial pleasure of that womblike wetness.

Sometime in 2000 he began climbing quietly out of bed every morning to pee on the floor. If we'd set the alarm for 5 a.m. and forced him to go to the bathroom, we might have caught him, but years of sleep deprivation still loomed large in our minds, eliminating that tactic.

One morning we heard Cam stirring and scurried into his room to find him poised on the edge of the bed, a puddle at his feet.

"Buddy! Don't pee on the floor; look what a mess you made!"

He looked up at us—the boy who seldom said anything intelligible—blinked and replied clearly, "I didn't know." Leslie and I exchanged wide-eyed looks.

She answered, "You did too know. We've only told you that a hundred times."

For a moment, it was as if we had a regular kid, and without thinking we'd responded as though he were one. Was he just offering the kind of feeble excuse other kids give when they do something they know they shouldn't have? Was he trying to explain that he'd been half asleep? Did he really not recall the countless reminders not to urinate on the floor? Why, then, did he act so guilty whenever we caught him doing it? But what if he meant exactly what he'd said—he hadn't even realized he'd urinated? A light shined onto the dark battlefield: was it possible that Cam didn't recognize the connection between the action and the consequence?

Eventually we just threw up our hands and arrived at a truce: we said nothing when he peed in the car or in the bed but kept the flow in check everywhere else. We bought a new living room rug and sofa and, through constant vigilance, managed to keep them nearly stain-free.

Clearly there was something deeply gratifying to Cam about the act of urinating. But the problem was knottier than that. People with autism often have neuromotor problems: they sometimes can't make their muscles obey them or don't recognize the signals their bodies send. Maybe Cam couldn't always sense when it was time to urinate until the feeling was so urgent that he couldn't restrain himself. And just as certain sounds that wouldn't bother you or me seem unbearably loud to him, perhaps his system intensified the full bladder feeling so much that he couldn't endure it even for a moment.

Then there's the sequencing problem. When you think about it, learning to urinate in a socially acceptable way involves a whole lot of motor planning. First you feel the sensation, and then you walk (or run) to the bathroom, where you pull down your pants, stand in the right place, aim carefully, and finally whiz into the water until you're finished. But you're not really finished: you still have to pull up your pants, flush the toilet, wash and dry your hands, put the towel back, and leave the bathroom. Cam has a severe "executive dysfunction"—an inability to sequence and carry out multiple-step actions. Many times he'd go into the bathroom and start peeing before he'd dropped his pants. Afterward, he'd sometimes walk away without pulling them up, or flush the toilet before urinating, or dry his hands before washing them. This set of tasks seemed impossibly complicated, and he acted as if he had to relearn them every day. Imagine if each visit to the toilet was like remembering a new set of dance steps. Would you perform them correctly every time? Would you bother trying?

But sensory and executive functioning problems don't tell the whole story. Throughout his life, Cam has had to find ways to compensate for his inability to speak. And he learned very early that when you let that pee go, adults jerk to attention. "So what if they're yelling? At least they're looking at me!" Urination gave him power he couldn't gain any other way.

Sometimes he exercised this power blatantly—"If I pee in the bed, I get to get up!"—but often he was more subtle. For example, upon arriving at his weekly gymnastics lesson, the first thing we'd do was go to the bathroom. The main reason was to prevent accidents, but retreating to this quiet place also gave Cam a moment to get his bearings and separate himself from the disorienting buzz and blur of the busy gym. In this case, his urination "problem" provided a way to calm himself and prevent blowups.

More often, however, peeing was a way to communicate. And he learned to say many, many things in this tongue, ranging from "I'm so anxious that I can't stand it" or "I'm confused and hurt" or "I'll show you!" to the obvious: "Boy, am I pissed off!" Alas, the flexibility of this liquid language was also its fatal flaw: since peeing could mean so many things, we never knew exactly what he was saying. Often we concluded that it didn't mean anything except that we *weren't* communicating. Sometimes it seemed that urinating had become an autonomous entity separate from him, that whatever message it conveyed wasn't even Cam's but that of the urine itself, speaking through him: "I'm peeing because that's what I do!"

Still, certain messages were hard to misinterpret. For instance, at the end of a rare summer afternoon when Cam and I had visited the mall, ridden the escalators, and shared ice cream, he was calm enough to sit in his room and listen to music. I was reluctant to bother him, but after forty-five minutes of tranquility, I went to his room to discover that he'd wet his bed. This was his little nudge to Dad: "You weren't noticing me." A little later he peed on the living room table and rug—just in case I'd forgotten.

Other times the message was clear only after the fact. For instance, one day he got off the bus wearing someone else's sweat pants, which meant he'd had a wet day at school. During his after-school work session, he wet his pants three more times. Ten minutes after we put him down for the night, he wet the bed again. For the three-hundredth time I explained, "Cam, you need to get up *before* you pee the bed. When you wet the bed, it makes the blankets yucky, and Mom and Dad have to wash them all the time."

He gazed at me for a few seconds until his brown eyes began their habitual wandering. "Anyway, wetting your pants and bed is what babies do. You're way too big for that. When you have to pee, *get out of bed.* You can do it, 'cause you're a big boy." I patted his head and left the room, pleased with the way I'd handled it. Heck, we might even have a dry night.

Les and I settled in to watch a hospital documentary. Engrossed in its moving true-life tales, we forgot about Cam for a few minutes. Then we heard tell-tale thumping from his room. Les shouted from his room, "He peed the bed again!" So much for my theory.

Then I remembered that the school nurse had told me one of Cam's classmates had slapped him during recess. Doubtless Cam had been saying in Urinish, "I'm scared 'cause a boy at school hit me." This time he'd been trying get attention and sympathy the only way he knew how.

But what about the hundreds of other times?

Often his emotions were clear, but his motives obscure. For instance, on one Saturday drive when Cam was eleven, he suddenly grew agitated and started shouting, "Hone, hone!" Dismayed that we didn't immediately transport ourselves to our driveway, he began to kick Leslie's seat and my shoulder, then pinched her arm hard enough to break the skin. Blood trickled from the wound as she tried to soothe him: "Okay, buddy, we're on the way home. Just hang on!"

As Cam rocked, growled, and kicked, I ran stop signs and broke speed limits. Les and I were literally sitting on the edge of our seats. By the time we pulled into our carport fifteen minutes later, our son was shrieking and thrashing like a man riddled with electric shocks. I yanked open the door. He wouldn't get out.

"Get out of the car," I commanded. "You were *bad,* so you need to go to your room." Right: if you knew you were going to be punished, would you cooperate?

I pulled him out of the seat; he went to his knees in passive resistance. I managed to lift him by the shoulders and march him toward the front door, but after a few strides he collapsed again. A neighbor living a few houses up the road stopped mowing his grass and gaped at the drama unfolding in our driveway: was this child abuse? Some bizarre game?

We stood uncertainly for a few minutes, waiting for Cam to calm down. Suddenly he sprang up, bellowed, slapped Leslie's head, and fell to his knees again. Enough! She picked up Cam's feet, I grabbed him behind the shoulders, and we hauled him like a casualty of war into the house, tossed him onto his bed, slammed and locked his door.

We stood there, faces flushed, hearts thumping, her arm bleeding, my shoulder aching. I stumbled into the den and stared at nothing for several minutes. The white walls seemed to pulsate. I felt as if I were suffocating.

As Cam bellowed, pounded on his door, and stomped his feet, Leslie sat beside me on the dark red love seat and began to weep.

"How long can we keep this up?" she asked between sobs.

"I don't know. As long as we have to, I guess."

After Cam grew quiet, I entered his room: he'd urinated all over the floor. But was he mad *because* he'd needed to pee, or had he peed to vent his fury? Had he, for some reason, *not* wanted to pee in the car, and so was enraged when he couldn't make us go home faster? Or was he already mad about something and using urine as an exclamation point?

For many minutes I mulled over these questions. I made no headway. I did know three things: (a) my son was imprisoned by his disorder, (b) Les and I were prisoners too, and (c) we all felt like warm piss.

But if Cameron was at the mercy of his excretory functions, the opposite was also true: he used urination to assert his will. He was determined to pee when and where he wanted to pee and prove that we couldn't stop him. Urinating gave him control not only over us but over a body that would not obey his other commands. No wonder he cleaved to it like a security blanket. He had created his own liquid language. Caught up in our own expectations and anxieties and determined to make him change, we couldn't comprehend his meaning. In a sense, we were as autistic as he was.

But though Cam was fluent in Urinish, it was a language even the fellow residents of Urinetown didn't understand. And if this habit separated us from friends and neighbors, it isolated my son most of all, leaving him alone in a world of sensations and meanings that nobody could share, not even those who loved him most.

Yes, the Martian is right: everyone's pain has a different smell.

Chapter 12

The Play of Shadows

I have a little shadow that goes in and out with me
And what can be the use of him is more than I can see
He is very, very like me from the heels up to the head,
And I see him jump before me when I jump into my bed. . . .
He hasn't got a notion of how children ought to play
And can only make a fool of me in every sort of way . . .
—Robert Louis Stevenson, "My Shadow"

A boy's room is a snapshot of his life and loves; the picture changes as he grows and gains new interests. And so my baseball cards and battered glove gave way to a stereo, Beatles posters, and orange paisley wall hangings.

Cam's room reveals his nature, as I discover one day when David, a man from Disability Services, visits to determine whether Cam qualifies for assistance. As we enter my son's bedroom, I suddenly see the room through a stranger's eyes.

"Wow, look at all the toys," David comments. A plastic Fisher-Price basket-ball hoop and backboard lean against the closet. A silver portable Sony CD player sits on the white nightstand; inside, CDs are piled helter-skelter, mixed with a heap of mutilated toddler books—*Goodnight Moon, The Runaway Bunny, Max's Christmas.*

Assorted children's videos—*Raffi in Concert,* Disney sing-alongs ("The Bare Necessities," "You Can Fly"), numerous *Kidsongs* tapes—spill over the top of a blue plastic trash basket; some lie on the floor. A giant blue therapy ball rests beside the twin bed. Beneath the window, a hulking trunk is packed with colorful toys: three different guitars, a "Magic Lights" keyboard, a new-looking baseball glove, two kid-sized basketballs, a Pinpressions novelty, a little boy's pounding bench. There are no other books, no video games, craft supplies, or soiled jerseys.

"How old did you say Cameron is?" David asks.

"Eleven."

I open the closet. Here lie the remains of six years of ABA therapy: bins of colored objects shine gamely into the darkness; twelve-piece puzzles, certain pieces chewed, are stacked unevenly on an aluminum bookshelf; above them, a Mr. Potato Head—nose twisted, tongue protruding, one arm gnawed to a stump—stares blankly. On the top shelf reposes a snazzy maroon bicycle helmet with dark brown flames running front to back.

Both of us remark the room's most striking feature: its stark white walls, which bear no garish hangings, no posters of pop stars or athletes. They bespeak a bare imagination, a boy who doesn't have heroes because he doesn't imagine being anyone else.

This is the room of a boy who doesn't play.

In this regard, Cam is typical of people with autism because the absence of imaginative play is one of the disorder's three distinguishing features. This impairment may not seem as debilitating as, say, the inability to speak, but it may be worse. For one thing, as Clara Park points out, an incapacity to play imaginatively seems to violate a fundamental human trait. No play means no curiosity and hence no science, no literature, no exploration—none of that vital élan that has raised humans from the mire. More concretely, the inability to play prevents autistic children from developing problem-solving skills, learning social cues, and hewing out the building blocks of other cognitive processes. Because play is, as Bryna Siegel puts it, the child's laboratory "for conducting 'experiments' on the things around him," a child who can't play doesn't discover novelties, expand his reach, or learn from mistakes. Hence, Siegel writes, "teaching a child with autism how to 'play' is tantamount to teaching the child . . . how to learn."

I explain to David that one of the main goals of our Lovaas program is to teach our son to play and imitate others. Under precise and limited circumstances, he can imitate certain gestures and facial expressions, but the larger goal—inducing him to interact with others—remains elusive.

I tell David how Cam learned the "Perfection" game (a matching exercise) well enough to match every one of its thirty squares to identical icons. I recall how Les and I watched, surprised and delighted, as Cam mastered a toy cash register, amusement park, and Fisher-Price car garage. But his mastery lacked creativity: he never pretended to hand out change or made those growly engine noises most boys can produce. His play remained as mechanical as the toys. He rarely used the skills outside of sessions, and novelty prompted resistance or downright hostility.

David assures me that my son qualifies for services. After he leaves, I finger the objects in Cam's room, each one embodying a failed attempt to spark his imagination. It is hard not to see them as monuments to dashed hopes. But then I realize that they are better seen as a material record of our relationship.

Chords Lost and Found

As a kid, whenever I wasn't reading, I was either playing or listening to music, riding my bike, or playing baseball. Our family was musical: my dad had a long-time country band, my mother sang in a well-regarded gospel trio, and they owned tons of records. I started piano lessons at age eight and have performed professionally throughout my adulthood.

Naturally, I pounced on any signs of musical interest in my son. They weren't hard to find. By age two, he was obsessed with music cassettes (everything from *Peter and the Wolf* to Pete Seeger) and sing-along videos. One favorite was "This Old Man." Thank heavens for the old coot! In moments of severe stress—at the dentist's office, waiting at the grocery checkout—Les and I could break into the song and Cam, no matter how anxious or upset, would join in—"This old man came . . ." "Roaning hone!"—and instantly calm down.

Dumbo's "If I See an Elephant Fly," *Pinocchio*'s "I've Got No Strings on Me," Raffi's "Baby Beluga," "Down by the Bay"—these songs have been the soundtrack of our life with autism. When Cam first started watching the Raffi videos, the children in the video audience were older than he was. They stayed the same as he grew bigger and bigger. To Les and me—and maybe for Cam—Raffi represents the early, happier years when Cam's cognition and senses were less disordered.

Favorites also emerged among the Disney videos, mostly exuberant tunes like "Mr. Toad's Wild Ride" (with its "merrily, merrily, merrily" chorus), "Supercalifragilisticexpialidocious," and "The Unbirthday Song." The films themselves bored Cam, but *Pinocchio* and *Dumbo* carried a special poignancy for his parents. We wondered: did Cam see himself in the gullible marionette who longs to be a real boy? Did he ever feel like Dumbo, oppressed by his muteness and shunned for his difference? Was his apparent lack of interest in the stories actually revulsion at witnessing his own disabilities portrayed?

He did watch one movie all the way through: *Mary Poppins*. He watched it every night. I mean *every* night. If we tried to interest him in a different movie, he vehemently insisted on "Poppins." It's a great movie; but even so, after the five-hundredth time, I swore that if I heard "A Spoonful of Sugar" one more time I'd surely upchuck.

It seemed plausible that Cam might want to play an instrument. When he was about six, I laboriously taught him a one-finger version of "Twinkle, Twinkle, Little Star" on the piano. I'd pull out his index finger (he couldn't point on his own) and strike the first note. We'd pound away roughly, my hand moving his reluctant pointer to the C, the G, the A, and so on. By the time we struck the last "are" he'd be squirming.

"Good playing, Cam! Want to play something else?" But he'd already be bouncing on his trampoline. Whenever I tried to show him a different tune, he insisted on "Twinkle, Twinkle"; if I persisted, he'd pinch me or run away. I later bought a programmable electronic keyboard with keys that lit up to show the melody; but the keyboard lit no spark in Cam.

At about age ten, he became fascinated with simple electronic musical toys. We bought all we could find, and he soon progressed from one-button toys to complicated guitars and keyboards. So what if the toys were designed for kids half his age—our son was playing!

We hit the jackpot with a *Blue's Clues* radio, a tiny toy with buttons that played six songs from the TV show. Cam had never watched *Blue's Clues,* but that didn't matter. What did matter was that (a) he liked the songs; (b) he could play an entire tune just by pressing one button; and (c) he could *choose* which one to play. There was a birthday song and a mail-time song, but Cam's number-one hit was the Solar System song: "Well, the sun's a hot star / Mercury's hot too / Venus is the brightest planet / Earth's home to me and you," all the way out to Pluto. For a couple of months, the toy was Cam's own satellite, perpetually orbiting him at arm's length.

One Saturday at the grocery store, while Les and I stopped to discuss lunch meat, our son, *Blue's Clues* radio clutched in his hand, slipped away. For fifteen seconds neither of us noticed his absence, then we fanned out in search of the lost boy.

I listened intently for his telltale laughs or shrieks. Instead, from a couple of aisles over, I heard, "Well, the sun's a hot star / Mercury's hot, too. . . ." In the soda aisle, his right hand gripping a large bottle of cherry seltzer, left hand grasping his radio, his chin turned to the ceiling, my son giggled and spun. Two middle-aged ladies gaped nearby, their shoulders hunched, afraid to approach the whirling body.

A few weeks later he threw the toy down and never picked it up again.

One Christmas my mother bought Cam a harmonica. This was better than a piano: you didn't need fingers, didn't need help. You just breathed and notes came out. For several weeks, the first thing he did after waking was pick up the "'monica" and blow a lusty "wheee—heee—heee." After a couple of huffs, he'd eagerly turn to me for approval.

"Good blowing, Cam! That's excellent!" He'd smile, sway, and clap.

We began presenting the harmonica as an activity and reward in the Lovaas program. But as soon as play became work, the harmonica was tainted, and Cam abandoned it. But one day months later, as he rummaged through the kitchen drawer where we kept stray toys, he spotted the harmonica and pulled it out. Putting it to his lips, Cam blew a loud chord.

"I sound good," he announced, shoving it back into the drawer.

The Cycle Cycle

As a tyke, Cam loved riding his stroller. He seemed to feel both protected and free while on wheels. When he was six, the Timberland staff told us he'd been riding a large tricycle at recess, so that Christmas we bought him an expensive black bike, complete with hand brake and training wheels. In the months that followed, we frequently took Cam and the bike out to the road beside our house. While I walked next to him, Les stationed herself fifty yards away, where the road reached a dead end.

"Cam! Ride to mommy!" she shouted.

As I held the bike, Cam carefully placed himself on the seat and stared down at the pedals. "Look where you're going, buddy, not at the pedals!" I pointed to his mom up the road. His head snapped up, but then he forgot to pedal.

I pulled the handlebars. "Come on, let's go fast!" He pedaled tentatively, with me giving frequent pushes, until we reached his waiting mom. "Way to go, Cam!" she'd shout, giving him a big hug. "You are so talented!"

Then we'd turn him around—making sure to keep him on the bike so he wouldn't be distracted by the weeds at the edge of the pavement or the smell of his mother's hair and forget about riding.

Within a month or so, he could ride the two blocks to the dead-end without crashing. The bike had replaced Cam's beloved stroller, literally: whenever he wanted to ride, he'd shout, "'troller!"

We were overjoyed: for once his abilities and interests were age-appropriate! But this budding skill presented a problem: Cam was big enough to ride at a rapid clip but lacked all sense of danger, and the return trip from the dead-end was all downhill. That meant he could pedal faster than I could run. And although I'd shown him how to brake countless times, he could never remember how when he needed to. I'd yell, "Cam, use the brake!" Thighs aching and heart thumping, I'd dash after him and grab the handlebars, usually just as he was about to slam into the curb or a parked car.

Once I slipped and Cam got away. As he streaked down the middle of the street, I stood, shoulders raised, teeth clenched, braced for an imminent crash.

"Buddy!" Les shouted, sprinting past me.

Luckily, the road runs uphill for thirty yards past our house, so gradually the bike slowed down, permitting Les to block it and halt our red-cheeked son.

After some months, however, he stopped requesting "'troller." Maybe he was frustrated that he couldn't get beyond the rudiments: a full year after we'd started, he still needed training wheels and couldn't consistently stop. Or maybe the whole exercise seemed pointless; unlike his dad, who, as a kid, rode his black Schwinn everywhere, Cam seemed to have no notion that the bike could take him places. And, frankly, we didn't want him to. If he left our sight, there was no telling what might occur; I was afraid even to imagine the horrible scenarios.

One day during the Late Bicycle Period, Cam's feet slipped from the pedals as he glided down the hill in front of our house. "Turn left! Turn left!" I shouted.

The black bike slowed, swung in a sharp spiral, and collapsed in a heap. Cam fell off, striking his penis on the seat. I ran to where he lay sprawled on the asphalt. "Doodle man! Are you okay?" He growled and slapped at my shoulder.

The bike was now toxic. He had learned an important fact: you could get hurt on that thing. By 1998 we'd given it away.

That Christmas, Cam disdainfully surveyed the presents under the tree, then turned to Leslie and said, "Stroller?"

She and I exchanged mystified looks. Cam clarified: "I need a present."

Somewhere he'd learned that boys got bikes for Christmas. Obviously, we were depriving our child of the one thing he really wanted. The next week we bought him a new bike. He wouldn't even get on it.

Thus ended the cycle cycle.

Strike Three

My sister and I grew up in a kid-filled neighborhood with two vacant lots that served as ball fields. When our gang wasn't playing baseball, I conducted imaginary games in our backyard. For hours on end, I'd hit and catch fungoes or sling the ball against the shed while pretending to be a major leaguer. I idolized ballplayers and collected hundreds of baseball cards, which I pored over, categorized, stacked, and filed daily. I knew every player's stats and wowed adults with this arcane knowledge.

When Cam was five I bought him a Wiffle T-ball setup.

"Okay, Cambo, let's hit the ball. Like this."

I put his hands on the bat, covered his hands with mine, pulled back the bat and took a healthy hack. "Now you do it."

He dropped the bat and ran away. I coaxed him to try again, this time keeping my hands on his as we walloped the Wiffle ball.

"Wow! What a hit! Now run!" He had no trouble with that part and generally dashed into the neighbors' woods.

The game must have seemed absurd: you run around to where you started, and then begin again. So why run? The notion of competing and winning was either beyond him—perhaps because it demanded that he imagine somebody else's thoughts—or seemed silly. Besides, he had his *own* rules: outside is for swinging or stripping bushes. Everything else is wrong.

I desperately wanted Cam to succeed at this, so every spring and summer we worked on hitting. He learned to hit a pitched Wiffle ball pretty well for an autistic kid, but he didn't *want* to hit the ball. I persisted, and when he was nine I enrolled him in a challenger league for disabled kids. At the first practice we waited for the coaches to get organized, which allowed ample time for Cam to move from his first base—reluctant cooperation—to second—wandering away, sitting down, plucking grass.

"Okay, let's hit the ball." I steered him toward the line forming near the batter's box.

"Huh-uh-huh-uh-huh-uh." He twisted his T-shirt in his fist and chewed on it, meanwhile gouging my knuckles with his nails.

Les questioned me with her eyes: is this worth it? I ignored her, then watched the other kids—Down syndrome girls and boys, kids with CP—whiff or feebly tap the ball. My boy could do better than that! But by the time Cam's turn to bat arrived, he'd mentally reached third base: angry defiance. Slumping to his knees in the muddy batter's box, he slapped the ground and growled. He refused to get up.

Red-faced, I implored, "Come on, buddy, I know you can do it. Don't you want to hit the ball? It's fun!"

"Wallace, this is not working."

"Let's just try it one more time."

"Mark. Think. This is ridiculous. Somebody's going to get hurt."

I stood, arms akimbo, a petulant ten-year-old whose mother has called him home from a game. Cam grabbed my T-shirt, ripped it, then sprang up and loped toward the car. Glaring at his back, I trudged in his wake. My kid had made a scene again. Christ, he couldn't even hold his own among other disabled kids!

Cam seemed to sense my intense desire for him to succeed, which burdened the game with expectations he couldn't (or didn't want to) meet. From then on, he went on a sit-down strike or fled as soon as I picked up the bat. In fact, swinging the Wiffle bat became a surefire way to get him into the house. I kept trying until one day, as I was chasing Cam around the yard holding the bat, I remembered how my own father had, despite my thick glasses, thin build, and obvious lack of enthusiasm, insisted that I try out for freshman football. At that moment I saw myself as another sports-crazed dad who hounds his son to live out unfulfilled dreams. I could almost hear myself shout, "Have fun, damn it!"

A Boy's Best Friend

Les and I came from dog families. Her family had two beagles, then a grubby Chesapeake; we owned a fidgety little mutt named Snooky, then a Lab-Irish Setter cross that my golf-besotted father named (against our vehement protests) Par. Snooky often followed me partway to school, barking as she turned back as if to remind me to keep my shoes tied and my nose blown.

Would a dog be a companion for our solitary son? In theory, maybe; but Cam didn't trust these wiggly, noisy, stinky creatures. By the time he was seven or eight, we could coax him to approach the neighbors' greyhounds and gingerly touch their coats. But all that ended one November Saturday in 1999.

That day, as Cam foraged around the yard, a neighbor boy happened by, walking two small, energetic black and tan mongrels. Seeing Cam, the dogs jerked free of their leashes and began barking fiercely. Then they charged. Cam's loping gait made him an easy target for the lead dog, who nipped at his shoes and legs as if my son were an errant sheep.

"Eeehhh!" Cam screamed, running in a circle and raising his arms as if about to take flight.

I stood staring for several seconds before sprinting down the hill to chase the dogs away. I scolded the kid, sent him home, then examined my son. The dog had bitten through Cam's jeans in two spots, but I didn't see any marks on him. No big deal: a near miss.

But when I returned from the bookstore ninety minutes later, the situation had changed dramatically.

The dog *had* broken Cam's skin. Les had called animal control; they'd urged her to phone the police. A policeman visited and told her to contact the owner, a neighbor we'd never met.

The conversation went like this.

"Hello. This is Leslie Gilden, from down the street."

"Oh, hello."

"I need to tell you that one of your dogs bit my son." She filled in the details.

"Our dogs don't bite. Your son must have teased him."

"My son is autistic and mentally handicapped. He isn't capable of teasing a dog." Her voice grew tight. "He was minding his own business, when your dog got away from the boy who was walking it and bit my son."

"The boy wasn't supposed to be walking the dog. Anyway, my dog wouldn't bite."

"Let me be clear: your dog attacked my *handicapped* son while he was *playing in his own yard.*"

"Oh, the dog might have snapped at him. That's how we play with them: we get them to snap at toys."

Silence.

"Well, I guess it's hard to understand."

"All I know is that your dog bit my son. We need to know if his rabies shots are up to date. We'd appreciate it if you'd check on that. We'll call you tomorrow."

The animal's shots were not up to date, which meant he had to be quarantined for ten days. If rabid, he'd be destroyed and Cam would have to undergo a series of painful shots. I grimaced as I envisioned the long needle puncturing his stomach.

During the quarantine, I battled guilt. I should have watched Cam more closely. I should have sensed danger and put myself between the dogs and my son. If Cam got rabies, I would never, ever forgive myself.

Fortunately, the dog was not rabid. But ever since, Cam won't go near dogs.

Cam's best friend (the only friend he has ever had) was not a canine but a human—another autistic boy named Andrew. I witnessed the friendship's birth one morning a few months later, when a slender boy with curly brown hair and sparkling dark eyes began to follow my son around. When Cam got on the slide, Andrew got on the slide; when Cam clapped, Andrew clapped; when Cam jumped on the tramp, Andrew jumped on the tramp. He was Cam's shadow.

The boys became inseparable at school. Outside of school, however, the relationship was hard to sustain. In fact, it seemed jinxed. Once Andrew's parents invited us to the Laurel racetrack for their son's birthday party. But an ice storm struck that day, making the forty-five minute drive too hazardous. Over the next few months, whenever we tried to arrange a play date, Andrew's parents couldn't commit or one of the boys got sick.

When summer school started the next year, Cam moved up to middle school, leaving Andrew behind. The friendship withered. Only later did I grasp what this meant.

As we were finishing a gymnastics lesson about a year later, Andrew unexpectedly walked through the door of the cool-down gym.

"Hey, Cam. It's Andrew. Hi, Andrew!" I said.

Andrew emitted a high-pitched squeal and trotted up to Cam. The boys exchanged double high-fives, clasped hands, touched foreheads. Andrew squealed again; Cam broke into giggles.

The pals had missed each other.

I'd never before seen my son acknowledge another child, let alone interact with one. Cam had been swinging in the middle of the room; now he gave up his seat for Andrew.

On the drive home that day I grew angry at the school all over again for separating the boys. They hadn't considered their friendship before making the change. Cam had reached the age to move, so they'd moved him.

Still, the relationship mystified me. Other boys bond over skateboards, video games, or card collections. But Cam and Andrew—both autistically self-involved—could hardly share interests. Did they recognize their common disability? Did my son, a head taller and fifteen pounds heavier, protect Andrew? Did he copy him? Did Andrew, with greater initiative and fewer problem behaviors, watch out for Cam? Was some mentor-protégé relationship taking place?

The scene at the gym had showed that, like other boys their age who hit each other, make fart sounds with their hands, or pull goofy faces, these two didn't need words to communicate. They simply enjoyed each other's company. They might have been friends even if they hadn't shared a disorder.

Why hadn't we done more to encourage this friendship? Maybe we simply couldn't believe that our son, who had always ignored other kids or treated them as nuisances, really had a buddy, a mirror in whom he could see and define himself. But perhaps there was another reason.

Me and My Shadow

We wanted Cam to learn to play so he'd have something to share with others. We wanted him to have the kind of experiences that had defined our childhoods. But maybe the reason I didn't do more to encourage his friendship with Andrew is that I didn't just want Cam to play; I wanted him to play *with me*. I wanted him to respond to my coaching, pedal beside me while I warned him about dogs and traffic lights. I wanted him to be my shadow, and he wanted to be someone else.

We've played two games together successfully, and neither carries memories from my childhood. When I cared less, he cared more.

One is hide-and-seek. In our version, I tickle Cam, then crouch behind a door. "Where's Daddy?" I ask. His eyes sparkling, his mouth twisted into the lopsided grin that means he's expecting something uproarious, he trots toward my voice, stopping every couple of feet to giggle. I growl, pounce, tickle his ribs. Cam semi-resists, then flees or collapses in laughter.

No cargo of painful expectations weighs us down. And no sign of this game lingers in his room. It exists only in memories of glee.

One evening when Cam was driving us bonkers—running through the house, pounding on the floor and walls, shouting himself hoarse, giggling incessantly, burping compulsively—I banished my worn-out wife to our bedroom and coaxed the boy into playing basketball.

Hoops has always made sense to him: you put the ball into the basket. When I hit a shot, I yell "Two points!," then, "Cam's turn." During my shot, he lies on the bed, bounces on the tramp, or stares out the window, but at his turn he almost always gives his best effort.

Over the years, I'd taught him a simplified version of H-O-R-S-E, which I'd named "ABC." I shoot from the center, then he shoots from there: A. We move to one side for B, then to the other for C. I have to prompt him to take each shot and praise him profusely for each basket. Occasionally he gets really excited and shouts, without prompting, "Two points!" If he misses two or three consecutive shots, he'll chew his shirt or bite the ball. He wants to succeed.

This evening he was even less compliant than usual. But a challenge sparked his interest.

"Cam, stand over here by the night stand. Try to throw it in from here!" He walked to the far end of the room, took aim, and missed. Twice. The growling and chewing commenced.

"Buddy, you can do it. Take your time and try again!" He took aim and sank it.

"Yay, two points for Cam!" We slapped five—like any father and son shooting hoops at home.

The struggle to teach my son to play was a prism refracting my own childhood—of days devising solitary games with private rules, conjuring a second self who narrated my life and drove me to excel. When Cam came along, I tried to make *him* my shadow. Only when I turned down the spotlight of my hopes and dreams did I glimpse the boy my shadow hid.

Cam also has a second self. It emerges whenever a bright light shines at the proper angle, and he stops whatever he's doing to create shadows on the table, wall, or door. It's as if he's talking in sign language to some unseen interlocutor. His hands, usually so maladroit, suddenly acquire grace and elegance. He seems both surprised and gratified by these shadows, as if he both knows and doesn't know that he has made them. Perhaps the shapes appear to him as abstract art, all chiaroscuro and contrast, each one pure and self-contained—*from* him, yet not *of* him. The shadow moves when he does, yet changes unpredictably—one minute small and helpless, the next large and menacing—a companion whose actions mirror his own. Perhaps the shadow, peeping from behind the blinds of his perception, appeals to him as a sign from another world—the elusive home, that place where he truly belongs. Or maybe the shadow self assures him that he is, indeed, truly himself.

Chapter 13

A Brief History of Stims

The soul has Bandaged moments—
When too appalled to stir—
She feels some ghastly Fright come up
And stop to look at her. . . .

The soul has moments of Escape—
When, bursting all the doors—
She dances like a Bomb abroad,
And swings upon the Hours . . .
—Emily Dickinson

Creative Destruction

Cam's hands embody his autism. Large and powerful, with long, elegantly tapered fingers, they could be a guitar player's hands. Usually, though, they dangle from his arms like a yearling colt's gangling hooves. They betray no signs of labor, not a single callus. He can't show you three fingers. He can't even make a firm fist. They are handicapped.

Yet those hands show remarkable dexterity and creativity when it comes to destruction. With them he can pinch and scratch until he draws blood, pull out tufts of hair, and swiftly unravel a shirt, string, or blanket strand by strand.

His creative destruction ranges from the small disturbances typical of ordinary toddlers—broken dishes, spilled liquids, washcloths flushed down the toilet—to the kind of havoc only a big boy can wreak.

One week I went to Montana for a visit, leaving Leslie to supervise Cam by herself. While she thought he was peacefully listening to music, he destroyed an air purifier's electrical cord. When she made a hasty bathroom visit, he dumped the contents of a piggy bank down the kitchen sink and turned on the garbage disposal. The grinding roar of the machine's death throes prompted a panicked dash to the kitchen, where Les found Cam staring intently at the drain. When he couldn't extract the draw cord from the living room blinds, he wrestled a kitchen chair to the refrigerator, climbed on top to get the scissors from their tray, strode back to the living room, and deftly severed the cord. Then he pulled the cord apart, one fiber at a time.

Most often, though, Cam's hands weave those soul-insulating bandages clinicians call "self-stimulatory behaviors," or stims. This term covers a wide spectrum of repetitive behaviors, from hand flapping, self-injury, and stereotyped manipulation of objects ("stereotypies") to watching the same movie over and over ("perseveration") and echolalia (repeating a previously heard word or phrase). Actually, everyone stims. If you chew your nails, compulsively tap your foot, clench your jaw, flip your hair, or fiddle with your moustache, you are stimming. But typical people's tics lack the all-consuming power of autistic stims.

Cam is a first-class stimmer. The stims have passed through stages, each more obsessive than the last. First were the Rocking Epoch—when he couldn't sit in a chair without violently rocking it back and forth—and the Swinging Stage. Then came the Stacking Phase, when every liftable object had to be placed on top of some other object.

The most amusing was the Wastebasket Era, which combined the stacking fetish with a container fixation. During this phase (Cam was about five), he'd roam the house dumping out the contents of every wastebasket, then place one—a white plastic kitchen garbage can was his bin of choice—on the living room floor or coffee table. With an arm on each rim, he'd carefully lift his rump and lower himself into the basket. There he'd sit, butt-deep in the basket like a miniature contortionist, his limbs hanging like petals on a wilting flower. He'd rock the basket till it tipped over, then pull himself out and start again. And again. Then again. As he Cam grew, the baskets got tighter and tighter, so that when he tipped over, he had a tough time getting out. I'd have to brace a foot on one side and yank him out, like Bugs Bunny popping out Elmer Fudd after he's been jammed into a bucket.

In 1996, at the crest of the Wastebasket Wave, Cam received a unique Christmas present from my mother: a three-foot-tall, bright blue plastic trash can. Les and

I tittered at it. But when our son emerged from his room on Christmas morning and spotted the trash can sitting bashfully among the brightly colored packages, he confirmed that the gift—an insulting one for most kids ("What'd you get for Christmas?" "A wastebasket.")—was perfectly suited to its recipient.

But eventually he became too big for the smaller baskets and too heavy for the taller ones. Thus ended the Wastebasket Era.

As a toddler Cam often tried to eat maple leaves. Were they toxic? Our medical guide was no help. I test-munched a couple; they tasted a little like radicchio. For safety's sake, we made Cam go indoors whenever he tried to snack on them. Did he quit chewing the leaves? No—he just ended up spending most of that summer indoors.

When the habit blossomed into full-blown twig-stripping, we tried again to nip it, but our yard's eight trees and massive forsythia hedge offered too many temptations. When we redirected him, he'd just trot to another bush and start up again.

Operation Bush never varies: find a slender branch at least two feet long—making sure it's not too thorny, brittle, or limp—and snap it from the bush or tree. While holding your prize in one hand, run the other hand down the stem, stripping off all leaves and smaller limbs. Fling away the denuded stick. Forage around the yard, sampling the plants—here a holly, there a dogwood, everywhere a stalk of poke—and repeat ad infinitum. It's hours of fun!

This habit would be incredibly tedious to most folks, but sameness is what fuels Cam's engine. His face shows the mix of concentration and blissful detachment that a typical child would display while setting up model trains. It's serious *and* relaxing, each branch a small challenge, a task with a clear beginning, middle, and end. This stim we could not wipe out, so we tried to restrict it to the hedge: forsythia grows so fast that you can't hurt it.

By 2000, the back of our neighbors' yard had gone wild: saplings interlaced with honeysuckle, wild ivy, multiflora rose, and other trash plants grew thickly. Cam gravitated to this oasis, and I let him, figuring he was at least occupied and safe. The neighbors said they didn't mind, so long as he stayed in the thicket, but I felt awkward about it and usually allowed Cam only a few minutes of pleasure before herding him back to our yard.

Then they planted a garden patch. Around it they built a chicken-wire fence—to keep out rabbits, they explained.

One afternoon as Cam was performing shrub surgery, I sneaked into the house for a bathroom break. When I returned two minutes later, our next-door neighbor, Ray, a stocky guy in his late thirties, was hanging clothes on the line. Cam now stood in their wading pool, contentedly pouring water from a pitcher onto the grass.

Ray scolded him, "Don't pour the water outside of the pool!"

I raced over, ignored Cam's angry slaps, and brought him inside. A few minutes later Ray rang our doorbell.

"I would really appreciate it if you'd keep him from playing in the wading pool, especially when I'm not there. If something happened, I'd be responsible, even if I wasn't around at the time. I don't let the other kids in the neighborhood play there either." Ray's careful courteousness told me that he was barely containing his rage—that and his red ears and sweating brow.

"Okay, I understand."

"Also, the garden. The plants are starting to grow over the fence. We often see Cameron walking near it. We put a lot of man-hours into that, and we don't want the plants ruined."

"Of course not. I don't think he's interested in it. He didn't touch the tomatoes last year. But absolutely, I'll make sure he doesn't go after the plants."

When I later told Les about the encounter, she said, "Oh, you know they've been talking about it. They're really mad, I'll bet."

No doubt: Ray's controlled seething had been hard to miss. I imagined the conversations: "I wish they'd keep that kid out of our yard. Why don't they make him do something else?"

So we began taking Cam to a nearby playground, where he could gather and strip until he got sick of it. But the habit pushed aside virtually all other outdoor activities. As Cam's stims grew stronger, his range of interests—and ours—grew ever more narrow.

Cords Lost and Found

Yet these outdoor stims couldn't hold a candle to the indoor ones. Which brings us to the cords. Oh, the cords! Cameron has had a cord or string obsession since he was five. It's his "signature" stim.

For several years, curly phone cords obsessed him, and our purchase of a cordless phone only encouraged him to switch to electrical cords. To prevent him from electrocuting himself, we started buying cheap curly cords, which he'd manipulate for long spells (usually standing in the same spot behind the couch), stretching and measuring the last couple of feet of each end until the cord frayed. Sometimes he'd scissor off the tips when they became uncurled. He'd often cut off more than he wanted, then get upset because the cord was too short. With a pleading look on his face, he'd hold out the damaged cord to one of us.

"What do you want? Do you want me to fix it?"

"Pis ek!"

Soon the cords had a new name: "Pis eks."

The name seemed apt, for it did seem that Cam was trying to "fix" the cords: fascinated by the straight versus curl distinction, he worked fiercely to stretch and straighten them out. Gradually he developed an entire system: he chewed partly through each cord about halfway down its length, then sculpted a plastic string from it that he set against the curly part. Then he chewed them into chunks. After biting through the plastic shielding, he'd unravel the small plastic lines inside the cord, gnawing and pulling them until the slender copper wires within were unveiled.

Studying each cord with the steely concentration of a surgeon stitching up a patient, he didn't respond to his name or notice if you left the room. Some compelling mystery seemed to lie within. Each cord was novel enough to require a bit of ingenuity to expose its entrails, yet ultimately each was a problem with a predictable solution. The process soothed and insulated him—a bandage against the threatening surround.

Diane Ellison strongly disapproved of the habit and persuaded us to extinguish it.

On the first day of this experiment, at the regular time—right after a meal—Cam approached Les. "Pis ek." No answer. He tried again. "Co'd."

"There's no more cords, honey. Want to play ball? Come on, let's get the ball!"

"Co'd!"

"I'm sorry, sweetie. You can't have any more cords."

He concentrated hard, clenched his brows, and carefully intoned, "I yant a new co'd."

"That's really good talking, Cam. But there's no more cords."

"Co'd, co'd, co'd, co'd!" He swung at Les, who intercepted his hand and said, "Let's go read a book. Want to read a book?"

His mouth turned in a perfect upside-down U. "I yant a new co'd!" Tears dribbled down his cheeks. "Aaaaahhhhh! Ooobbbb!"

We held the line, so to speak, and pretty soon he stopped bawling and beseeching. We tried replacing the cords with an "appropriate" activity—a "lace 'n' trace" game. He just unraveled the yarn.

Then he began tearing covers or pages from books, ripping pages from my teaching notes, and chewing up the paper. Within a month, a good 10 percent of our books had been mutilated. Cam managed to strike us where it really hurt, and we couldn't help but wonder if this "stim" was designed to do just that: now he was "fixing" us. What better way to change our minds about the cords? The maimed books and chewed-up paper wads seemed far worse than the messy but innocuous cords, so after an agonized discussion, we gave him back the phone cords.

Cam's stims, we concluded, are like addictions. Instead of trying to go cold turkey, it was safer to put him on methadone. And if the phone cords gave him—and us!—a few minutes of tranquility, it seemed pointless to meddle. The habit did leave a trail of curly plastic strips on the floor that made our living room resemble a hair salon for electrical appliances; every evening one of us would sweep up, muttering curses about the pigsty we lived in. But it seemed a small price to pay for peace.

At the height of the Cord Craze, we were buying a dozen a week. Fortunately, the Dollar Store down the street carried cheap ones that readily yielded their guts to Cam's exams. During stock-ups, I'd feign nonchalance as I lifted the shopping basket overflowing with variously colored phone cords onto the checkout counter. The clerk would eye me quizzically, sometimes commenting, "You must have a lot of phones!"

I'd nod or say something noncommittal: "Oh, you can never have too many telephones."

The clerk would shake her head and half smile. She'd never have believed the truth.

Then the Phone Cord Phase took a dangerous turn. One afternoon, I noticed that Cam had chewed partway through the electrical cord running from his lamp to the wall socket. We immediately removed all lamps and electrical cords from his room; the next week we installed overhead track lighting.

A few days later, Cam chewed up our stereo speaker cords. I restrung them. The next day he tore them up again. I restrung them again. He ripped them up again. I drilled a hole in the floor and laboriously restrung the wires through the crawl space beneath, leaving only a foot of exposed wire between the hole and the speakers. When Amanda, his Lovaas therapist, arrived that day, I retired to my office, nursing a tiny sense of satisfaction.

An hour later I ventured upstairs to find Cam sprawled in a chair; Amanda knelt before him, trying to detach his hand from her hair. I glanced at the floor: there lay a shredded cord. Cam had destroyed the new speaker wire I'd just strung.

A red shade dropped over my eyes. "Cameron! What did you do?" I bellowed. Holding his chin in my right hand, I shouted, "Daddy just fixed these and you ruined them again! God damn it!"

My son stuffed his fingers into his ears and ducked into his room. Why was Daddy so mad? All he'd done was take apart a cord, something he'd done every day for years. Amanda wouldn't meet my eyes: this had happened on her watch.

Head pounding, I stomped outside, looking for something, anything, to hit. Snatching up the yellow Wiffle bat, I slammed it against a maple tree over and over until the bat splintered. If neighbor Ray had peeked over the hedge at that moment, his suspicions would have been confirmed. Our child stripped branches off trees; I was trying to chop one down with a Wiffle bat. What next?

I stalked around the yard fuming. At the tail end of a long summer when I'd been with Cam for several hours every day, my nerves were as frayed as one of his cords. We lived in a totalitarian state, slaves to Cam's obsessions. Now he was pulling off *my* bandages, too!

For the rest of the summer we listened to music through headphones, sealed into our private spaces. Our son had again reshaped our world to mirror his autistic domain.

In September I nailed sturdy, black speaker wires to the molding. Cam never noticed them. Our music was restored; even better, we had won a small victory over autism.

The String Thing

Eventually the cord fetish went away. Or rather, it mutated, as the ever-inventive mind of Cameron introduced New Improved Shredding and Tearing. His specialty: fabrics of all kinds, especially but not exclusively clothing.

At age six, he'd sometimes get off the school bus wearing only the top portion of an unraveled knit shirt, the vestiges hanging pathetically from his neck as if he'd burst through it like the Incredible Hulk. He forgot about this superpower—until 2000, when, out of nowhere, it returned with a vengeance, shouldering aside the phone cord fixation.

One by one Cam destroyed his T-shirts. His socks and underwear soon followed. We bought heavy shirts; he shredded them. We bought natty sweaters; he tore them up. At wit's end, Les dressed Cam in two of her old bulky sweaters. They deterred the tearing demon for most of the winter. Then the String Thing evolved again.

Within three days, Cam destroyed all five of his comforters, leaving intact only a blanket made from a synthetic material called Solaron. Les found online some similar blankets made of Polartec—soft material thicker than regular cloth. We selected the arctic blue and the sand at $79 each. "They're not cheap, but they should last awhile," we assured ourselves.

We oohed with satisfaction when the new blankets arrived and proudly showed Cam the new purchases. Les set him on the couch and wrapped him in the blue number. Snuggling down, Cam was the picture of warm contentment. Les and I retreated to the kitchen.

Seconds later: "Zzzzffttssssttszz." The now-familiar sound of ripping.

I followed it into the living room. My son had torn the new blanket almost in half. I opened my mouth to yell, then stopped and shrugged. What was the point? The blanket problem had been solved for approximately three minutes.

A few days later, we found more synthetic blankets at the neighborhood Wards. Because the material was elastic and stretched before it tore, Cam found it difficult to execute his master strokes of rending. He still tore them apart piece by piece—every morning we found more strips on the floor—but at least the demolition took awhile.

Over the next few months, he destroyed any shirt we put on him. By summer we were letting him go topless most of the time. And it wasn't just his own clothing: any laundry left within reach was soon rendered into confetti. He seemed fascinated by the process of reducing a whole to its component parts. Even more mesmerizing were the fibers themselves: smaller, more challenging versions of the cords.

Then one day, while watching Cam shred the laces on my sneakers, Les had a flash: maybe a shoestring would appease him. For the next few days, whenever he started to tear fabric, we gave him a flat, white shoestring. And so we arrived at the Shoestring Solution.

Here's how it works. Take a shoestring and extract several small threads, one by one. Pull on both ends of each thread, wrapping it around your fingers to create a taut band that twangs like a ukelele. Pluck at the tiny fibers until they become gossamer bits of fuzz. Then fling them away or blow each one into the air. Continue pulling strands, making sure to litter the floor. Repeat. Repeat. Repeat. Repeat. Repeat. Repeat. Repeat. Repeat. When you've created a wad of strands, cram the whole thing into your mouth and chew it like gum.

Shoestrings, like phone cords, are made of a myriad of tiny filaments fascinatingly woven together, offering minute variations within a larger structure of sameness. Cam tolerates their minimal novelty—even welcomes it—because he knows the end of the story. Dwelling in his wonderland of strings, he makes his own quiet music.

When your child finds so little happiness, when he feels such pain, when he is barred from most human interaction and bereft of typical sources of joy, you don't have the heart to deny him his balms, no matter how strange they seem to you.

We can also use strings as rewards or enticements. But he's onto the trick, and sometimes resists it. For example, one day we bought Cam another bunch of new toys, but he still insisted on having a string. Then in one of my guilty phases, I decided that he should work for it.

"Do you want a string?"

"'Tring, yes."

"Then you need to play a song on your new keyboard. You have to *earn* your string."

Pinch, gouge. "Ahuh-ahuh-ahuh! 'Tring!"

Leslie poked her head into the room and frowned. What was I trying to prove?

"Do you want a string?"

"'Tring!"

"You need to play one song. Just one song."

My son twisted the front of my shirt. I pulled his fingers free; he studied my face for a few moments and decided I wasn't going to give in. With much growling and chomping on his "suckie," he chose "Old MacDonald," and grudgingly pushed the lighted keys one by one until he'd played the whole song.

Afterward he had to shout "Aaah aahhh, aahhh" and pound the walls in protest. But he had earned the string, and I felt vindicated: I hadn't lost my temper and I hadn't given in.

A couple of hours later, when he thought I wasn't listening, I heard him experimenting with the keyboard.

Bandaged Moments

The most confounding aspect of Cam's stims is this: though dexterous enough to pluck out the tiniest filaments of a shoelace, he can't draw a straight line or make a V sign.

Then there's the deeper mystery: why does he want to do the same thing over and over? Experts offer differing explanations. One theory is that stims are "secondary coping mechanisms"—responses to overarousal and anxiety. This is the motive given by autistic authors Temple Grandin and Donna Williams, who write that their stims allowed them to focus on something safe and familiar, thus furnishing the "bandaged moments" that Dickinson's poem describes. Stimming arrests the streaming world and renders it less threatening, permitting autists to weave for themselves a nice, comfortable cocoon.

Another view attributes stims to an impaired "theory of mind." This hypothesis holds that autistic people don't understand that other people have thoughts they themselves do not. According to this theory, an impoverished capacity to interact socially leaves autistic people little choice but to pursue isolated, repetitive actions. This explanation raises disturbing questions about what it means to be human. Most of us create ourselves in part through relationships, interpreting our selfhood through the reflections received from others, learning about ourselves by extrapolating from others' behavior. But autistic people are often mystified by other humans and instead develop relationships with objects. Does this tendency make them less human?

A third approach sees stims as evidence of that lack of "central coherence" I discussed earlier. In this view, because Cam's fragmented and unpredictable perception prevents him from placing objects and actions into wider contexts, he concentrates on minutiae. Strings provide *local coherence,* permitting him to make sense of at least one small fragment of his world. In the face of Cam's difficulties in creating workable theories about the world—he usually over- or undergeneralizes from specific experiences—strings offer compelling and predictable data. Like a cosmologist, he explains the world through string theory.

A fourth view sees stims as a symptom of executive dysfunction, which involves two separate disabilities: an impaired ability to stop actions once they're started (that familiar autistic perseveration) and an inability to begin novel actions. Cam can't change direction once he starts something and can't think of new things to do when he stops. One researcher suggests that the real problem isn't just an inability to translate goals into action but an inability to conceive of goals in the first place. Perhaps the causality is reversed: executive function deficits may result from the constant repetition of the same actions, which inhibit the generation of neuromotor skills needed to initiate novel actions.

Each of these has seemed accurate to us at different times. We've seen Cam beg for a string when he was upset or anxious, as one of us might pour a glass of wine; we've witnessed him stim to block out the din of a roomful of people; we've watched him stim when bored. Whatever the motive, stims let him fashion meaning from an incomprehensible world.

There is indeed a kind of purity—what Clara Park calls a "strange integrity"—in Cam's stims. He's like Whitman's "noiseless patient spider" on its promontory, launching filament after filament "till the ductile anchor hold." He is Robinson Crusoe on his island, building a private utopia with what's at hand. No one shares the island; he's unreachable, self-involved, impervious. Yet his ability to remake the world in his own image, to block out distractions, is quintessentially human. Ironically, his seemingly alien behaviors only reveal that Cam is really one of us.

Dancing Like a Bomb

From time to time, though, his soul explodes from its cocoon. Sometimes it happens when his body dances.

When he was four, Les would put on a record—Tina Turner's *Private Dancer* was a favorite—and for twenty minutes sway and spin around the room while holding Cam like bundle. She did this nightly for months, despite the herniated disk in her back and despite that fact that she weighed about 115 pounds and Cam weighed a good 50. Why? Because he loved it and because afterward he was markedly more relaxed and focused.

Cam still dances when he's happy: he slides his head from side from side to side, then back and forth like a pigeon when it walks; then he bends his knees, throws his hands back as if tossing sand, and springs into the air with a scissors kick. He lands with his head poised near his knees—a break-dancer caught in freeze-frame. It's graceful and ungainly all at once.

In fact, he has always loved to move through the air. At age three, he satisfied this craving with long bouts on his trampoline. The boy was a bouncy, flouncy, pouncy, jouncy human Tigger. Our occupational therapist informed us that this activity gave him "vestibular stimulation"—a function of the inner ear—which helped him determine where his body began and ended. The tramp sat in front of our picture window, and from there Cam could watch TV or listen to music as he leaped. We frequently found him stark naked, offering an intriguing spectacle for passersby. But nobody seemed to notice.

Once while out for a walk, Leslie met a woman she knew from work. The lady asked where we lived. When Les described our house, the woman's eyebrows went up: "Oh, where the naked boy lives!"

Okay, so someone *had* seen him.

Like most kids, Cam also loved to jump on his bed; like most parents, we prohibited it. Even so, we'd often hear him in his room at night, throwing himself back on the mattress again and again. One evening—he was about seven—the bouncing ended with a loud thump, then dead silence. We dashed into his room to discover Cam lying stunned and quivering, his face purple, his mouth contorted. He'd cracked his head on the wall. He was trying to wail but nothing would come out; the cry was being wrenched from so deep in his gut that he couldn't even shriek. We waited in mounting panic until he caught his breath, then gave forth torrents of choked screeches and sobs. The waves of ululation gained force: all the frustrations of his young life were concentrated in that cry. After a quarter hour, his howls abated, and a huge, tender knot rose on the back of his head.

We frantically thumbed through our medical guide for the symptoms of concussion and skull fracture. No, his pupils weren't unevenly dilated; no, he didn't seem dazed or sleepy—just very, very sore. Playing it safe, we took turns sitting by his bed all night, afraid to let him sleep (because sleeping with a concussion, we read, can sometimes induce a coma), yet knowing sleep was exactly what he needed

During my first shift, I gazed down at my son, hiccupping drowsily after his crying jag. Stroking his hair, I regarded the long lashes curling over his eyes. Why couldn't I protect him from himself?

Surely, you'd think, that was the end of his bed bouncing. You'd be wrong. Yes, we pulled him off the bed and scolded him whenever we caught him bouncing, but he so needed the feeling of being airborne that he couldn't help himself. At least he never again missed his aim.

Clinicians might call this a stim, but the line between playing and stimming can be blurry. For example, when Cam was between three and five he passed through a Climbing Craze. Yet climbing was only the means to his end, which was to get high—literally. After entering a room, he'd immediately head for the highest point, usually by clambering up on a table or couch. When he reached the top, he'd stand as proud and straight as if he'd just climbed K-2. His balance was remarkable: he never fell.

At six and seven, he switched to climbing our twin Japanese maples. He could nimbly scramble from the strong, low-hanging branches up into the middle of the tree. Roosting there, he'd gaze upon his domain, crowing and clapping loudly. He loved climbing so much that we used it as a reward following therapy sessions. Once he interrupted a session to announce, "I want to go outside and climb a tree." We immediately suspended work and obeyed his request. That sentence remains one of the longest he's ever uttered.

Is this playing or stimming?

One of Cam's favorite videos depicts Peter Pan convincing the Darlings that thinking of something happy is "the same as having wings." "You can fly!" he exclaims, and, to their amazement, they can. During Cam's Climbing Mania, my greatest fear was that he'd take Peter at his word; I entertained visions of my son springing from the tree, flapping his arms, and crashing to the ground.

Luckily that never happened, and eventually tree climbing yielded to a more controlled form of flight.

When Cam was three, we had an expensive wooden swing set built in our yard. It turned out to be the best investment we ever made. He spent some of his happiest hours there. Swinging furnished the vestibular stimulation of jumping or flying but with far less danger. For many years, swinging was virtually the only "normal" activity he'd willingly do outdoors. Sure, swinging was similar to autistic rocking. But it gave him exercise and provided a chance for us to play with him.

Wouldn't it be even better if he could swing on his own?

For years we tried to teach him this skill. "Put your legs out, Cam," I'd say. "Then when you swing back, put your feet back."

He stared somewhere near my shoulder.

"Come on, let's go! Out . . . and back. Out. . . . and back." His feet still dangled. "Try again. Out . . . and back. Out and back."

Cam joined in the chant: "Out," he echoed, voice rising at the end. "And bek!" His mouth soon had the rhythm down cold. His legs did not. Did he fail to understand that he needed to kick out, or couldn't he manage to give his legs the commands? Both?

After several months of futility, I tried a new tactic. Once I'd pushed him to a reasonable level, I'd hold out my palms and ask him to kick my hands. But he wouldn't continue for more than a few seconds after I dropped my hands.

These skills seem so rudimentary, so instinctive, that it's easy to forget how much motor planning is involved. You have to lean back, hang by your fingers, then kick toward the sky, which demands balance as well as strength. Then you must quickly shift your weight forward and bend your knees beneath the seat for the return trip. Such complex sequences baffled Cam. At age eight, he seemed no closer to swinging independently than he'd been at three. I tried one last gambit.

"Poosh," he begged.

"Daddy can't push. You have to swing by yourself."

"Swing!"

"You can swing by yourself, bud!" I walked away, ignoring the "Aaah, aaah, aaahs" that trailed me.

This went on for several weeks, until the swing set had become yet another source of anxiety. Les asked what I was trying to accomplish.

"Maybe if he realizes I won't help, he'll figure it out himself."

She shook her head. "He *can't* figure it out! Why are you torturing him!"

"We've tried everything else. And I'm sick of push, push, push!"

"You're still in denial, Wallace." This had become her usual response when I tried to push Cam beyond his capacities; she believed I couldn't accept the severity of his disability. In fact, I was just frustrated.

So I gave up. Though I still coached him with the "out . . . and back" chant, I was just, well, going through the motions.

A week later I took him outside to swing. "Poosh!" he begged.

"Okay, buddy, here's a push." I gave him a shove and stood with my arms folded. I'd be damned if I'd push him again. I grabbed the Wiffle bat and started hitting fungoes into the hedge.

After one hit sailed across the street, I turned to check on Cam. My son was flying high, his feet nearly touching the outer limbs of the tree. I gaped in astonishment as he kicked forward, tucked his knees backward, forward, then backward.

"Cam! You're swinging! You're swinging!"

He glanced at me briefly, then stared straight ahead: this was hard work.

"Yay, Cambo man! Look at you! You're going really high!"

His face broke into a wide smile. "Hah, hah, hah. Hee, hee, hee."

Had our years of hard work finally paid off? Or did he succeed only when I stopped trying so hard?

Cam's school day ended early on Wednesdays. To fill up these vacant afternoons, we launched our grandest experiment in play—gymnastics lessons.

At first he'd burrow deeply into the jumping pit (a box filled with foam rubber squares) and refuse to come out. Or he'd dash across the gym and interfere with the tots' tumbling classes or pilfer their sodas. But before long he eagerly looked forward to "nackets."

Not surprisingly, his favorite activity was jumping on the giant trampoline (it was placed at floor level and surrounded by pads, so it was pretty safe). Bridget, a slim German immigrant with a faint sing-song lilt to her English, was his coach. Persistent, gentle, and patient, she used the promise of the tramp to induce Cam to finish his warm-ups and try other activities.

He learned to do somersaults and perform a seat drop and knee drop, but most loved launching himself into the air. I'd watch with a mix of anxiety and admiration as my son fearlessly bounced higher and higher, turning in circles, an expression of untrammeled bliss on his face whose meaning was unmistakable: "I can fly!"

Cam's other favorite activities involve liquids. Whenever he sees a half-empty container, he *must* pour the liquid all out. Les jokes that for Cam all fluids have only one desire—to return to the mother source. They simply *cry* for release! After helplessly watching countless bottles of shampoo, detergent, contact lens solution, soda, juice, and cups of coffee disappear down the sink or bathtub, we learned to hide them.

The water fetish extended to the bathtub. During one period, Cam demanded four or five baths per day. This may seem a healthful habit. But he didn't take ordinary baths. No, he had to bite the soap—rare was the bar that didn't bear an impression of Cam's teeth—and fill a large blue cup (pocked with teeth marks) and pour it out again and again; he also had to divert the faucet's stream all over the room. The results? A flooded bathroom, piles of soggy towels in the corner; no hot water in the tank; and, eventually, a rotted wall and window.

Hoping to transpose this obsession into a different key, we started visiting my college's pool several times a week during the summers. But though Cam loved splashing around, he lacked the motor skills to swim. Les speculated that if we could bypass his brain, muscle memory might take over. So for one whole summer they worked on kicking. She'd place her hands on Cam's calves, say, "Kick your feet," push his legs down and up in a kicking motion, then heave him toward deep water. Nothing clicked.

One Saturday in 1998—at the end of a summer when Cam and his nanny had taken daily dips—the family went to the pool. Les helped Cam kick for awhile. Then, as she and I traded places, he pulled himself out of the water, ran toward the deep end, and plunged in at the eight-foot mark. I watched my son's head sink beneath the surface. My heart stopped; I couldn't move. Then the spell broke: I dived and swam frantically toward him. All of a sudden Cam popped up, giggled, and calmly paddled toward the side.

My wife was right: when he didn't think about what to do, he could get out of his own way. Over the next year, he developed his own peculiar stroke—a dog-paddle combined with a frog kick, performed while perpendicular to the surface. He appears to be walking in the water. But it works for him.

An alien environment for most of us, water feels like home to Cam. There are no rules to learn and nothing to manipulate. It's locally coherent: you sink or swim. Enveloped in the womb-like liquid, he finds himself again. Even better, he lets *us* find him, and sometimes even lets us share the shallows at the rim of his island.

In these moments, his soul bursts its doors, throws off its bandages, and dances like a bomb. In these moments—more glorious because so rare—we are all emancipated.

Chapter 14

As Others See Us

O wad some Power the giftie gie us,
To see oursels as others see us!
It wad frae many a blunder free us,
An' foolish notion . . .
—Robert Burns, "To a Louse"

Rain Man Moments

As we stand in the checkout line at the grocery store one Saturday, Cam snatches up the half-full soft drink of a middle-aged lady standing nearby. Leslie smiles apologetically. "I'm sorry," she says. "Cameron is autistic, and you've just experienced what we call a '*Rain Man* moment.'"

The lady returns her smile. "Oh, it's no problem. Don't worry about it."

"Knees up, Brown! Hoppin' on one foot!" Cam explains.

Les used the phrase because at the time the average person's knowledge of autism came from the movie *Rain Man,* in which Dustin Hoffman plays Raymond Babbitt, an autistic savant who can memorize half a phone book in a single night. Having lived in an institution for more than twenty years, Raymond is totally wedded to his routine—Judge Wapner at three, *Jeopardy!* at five, and lights out at eleven. When his arrogant younger brother Charlie kidnaps him, Raymond calms himself by reciting the Abbott and Costello routine "Who's on First." When Charlie tries to get him on an airplane, Raymond, convinced by TV news that air travel is unsafe, throws a head-slapping, shrieking public tantrum.

"No flying!" he screams.

"No flying, no flying," Charlie assures him.

Taking Cam out in public presented a similar dilemma. He needed to leave the house and learn to behave, and sometimes enjoyed watching other people. By the time he was ten, we'd developed an itinerary of tried-and-true places: the pool, gymnastics lessons, supermarkets and convenience stores, McDonald's or Burger King.

Even in familiar locations, however, Cam was unpredictable: some days he'd stroll happily beside us, sipping a Coke; other days he'd fall to his knees, destroy merchandise, shout and pound his chest, or start slapping at us. Each trip was an obstacle course. We'd make our way down the aisles, faking nonchalance, but in fact we were hypervigilant, eyes darting left and right for possible hazards—a balloon or string, a senior citizen eating a donut. We held our breaths until safely back in the car, then heaved sighs of relief.

Despite the stress of these excursions, they made us feel a little less like prisoners, so we'd worked out strategies to maintain safety: flank Cam, keep his hands occupied, tell him what came next, show him his picture schedule. But there were still plenty of *Rain Man* moments.

On the way home from the Giant that day I said to Leslie, "I would never explain to someone I don't know that Cam has autism. I would just tell him 'no' and apologize." I didn't want to share our lives with strangers, didn't want their indulgence or pity. Les's straightforward explanations seemed to me signs of weakness. No doubt my reticence was a form of denial: if I didn't ask for help, I could pretend that I wasn't the father of an autistic child.

But Les was right: taking people into your confidence deflects blame from your kid (or your own lousy parenting) and places it where it belongs—on the disorder. You bridge the gulf between the "normal" and "abnormal" by showing that you accept your child as he is.

Yet Cam's worst moments, like Raymond's, were impossible to explain away. He was now five feet tall and weighed a hundred pounds, so his outbursts weren't just curious, they were dangerous.

Crossing the parking lot by our regular swimming pool, Cam abruptly begins to slap me on the arms and shoulders. I hesitate: does he want to stop, or is he just eager to start swimming? Aware that he usually calms down once we get into the water, I ignore the blows and steer him toward the lounge chairs scattered around the cool blue water's rim. To our left, a young female lifeguard lies prone, eyes closed, soaking up sun. Suddenly I hear a loud "Yow!" Swiveling my head, I see Cam clutching a handful of the girl's long blonde hair.

I try to untangle his fingers. "Cam, let go now!" I try not to shout, but feel my face get hot. The girl, her head tilted at a severe angle, whimpers and taps vaguely at Cam's hands. His face shows no emotion, but he won't relinquish his hold. I sense the stares boring into our backs. At last I free his hands. "I'm sorry," I say. "He has autism and gets fixated on things."

"It's okay," she replies with a sniffle, patting her ruffled locks.

It is *not* okay. I thrust my fingers into the back of Cam's trunks and hustle him to the pool fence. In a stern stage whisper I scold him: "That was very bad! If you can't be good, we're going home right now!"

He regards me briefly, then looks away, his face expressionless. Does he understand? I consider taking him home, but we've already come this far, so we return to our lounge chairs and begin to disrobe. As soon as Cam's shirt and shoes are off, he lopes to the deep end and prepares to jump in. I tell him to wait for me because he can't swim well enough to jump in there.

He hops, slaps his chest, and growls. That's it: I grab him by the left arm and escort him, in a stumbling trot, back to the car. As I buckle him into the back seat, I feel an artery throb in my temple but hold my tongue, afraid I'll explode into animal roars if I open my mouth. I remain in teeth-gritted silence until I find my way to the driver's seat.

Then I bellow, "If you didn't want to go swimming, why did you say you wanted to? Shit!"

Cam kicks the back of my seat. "Shit!"

"Shut up!"

"Up! Ah, ah, ah, ah, ah!"

Too upset to find this funny, I stare grimly ahead, fingers gripping the steering wheel as my son screeches and kicks.

He's never before acted this way at the pool. What's wrong? A minute's pondering yields only a shrug: by this time I've concluded that many of his outbursts have no motive, but are just eruptions of the autism imp. Muttering into the wheel, I pull the car out of the lot.

As soon as we reach home, Cameron has a big bowel movement. I'm nearly as relieved as he is: this time his behavior has a logical explanation. But why hadn't told me needed to go, as he ordinarily does? Did he assume I knew he needed to poop? Was he afraid that if we crossed the road to the bathroom, he wouldn't get to swim? Maybe I overreacted. But am I expecting too much of him or not enough?

Aliens

In Cam's early years, we were painfully self-conscious: whenever he clapped or squealed in public, we blushed in embarrassment, feeling as though everyone could read the scarlet letter—A for autism—glowing on our chests. Eventually we grew thicker skins, and Cam's behavior came to seem more ordinary. Other people's reactions, however, reminded us that they regarded him differently.

We encountered well-meaning folks who knew enough to be sympathetic but seemed offended when Cam didn't acknowledge their generosity; a few others insinuated that his behavior was our fault and sometimes offered unsolicited advice ("Did you try saying 'No' to him?"). Occasionally we'd encounter people who worked with disabled kids, who'd say, "Oh, he's autistic, isn't he? Where does he go to school?" They seemed to want our approval, in return for which they could say, "You guys are so good with him." We learned to appreciate those who just looked the other way.

We became experts in parsing what disability scholar Rosemarie Garland-Thomson calls the "taxonomy of staring." There is the wondrous stare, which perceives the disabled person as a hero overcoming adversity; there is also the sentimental stare, which regards the person as a pitiable victim; and the exotic gaze, which renders the person strange and entertaining, yet irremediably alien. Last and least painful is the realistic stare, which acknowledges a connection between the starer and the person stared at. We experienced all of these at one time or another.

On our better days, we laughed it all off, quoting a scene from a favorite movie, *Invasion of the Body Snatchers,* when a doctor played by Kevin McCarthy and his female companion are fleeing from alien pod people who've just told them, "Tomorrow you'll be one of us." The two don't want to become robotic pseudo-humans, but to survive, they must pretend to be. McCarthy tells his friend, "Keep your eyes wide and blank. Show no emotion or excitement." Preparing for an outing, Les and I would often recite the lines, bug our eyes out, and walk around like stiff-legged zombies until we burst into giggles.

But on other days, I could barely suppress the urge to drop my jaw and gape back at the gapers. One Saturday at the supermarket, Cam made a dash for some balloons hanging near the produce section. A middle-aged lady and her chubby preteen daughter got an eyeful as Cam pulled off a ribbon, twirled and then shredded it. The two openly gawked, offering comments under their breath. My son was far more entertaining than the watermelons displayed nearby.

I flashed back to a scene from Tod Browning's *Freaks,* a movie about life in a circus sideshow. One regular-sized woman, a trapeze artist named Cleopatra, pretends to love a little person named Hans, though she's really after his money. During their wedding feast, the other performers serenade them:

>We accept her, one of us
>We accept her, one of us
>Gooble gobble gooble gobble
>One of us, one of us.

Quick cuts show us a bearded lady, several microcephalic people, and John-ny Eck, the famous legless performer. Finally the camera rests on Cleopatra, wearing a look of abject horror. One of *them*? Oh, God, no!

I opened my mouth, about to shout at the starers, "Step right up and take a gander. Hurry, hurry, hurry! Behold the freak of nature! If you come closer you can even feed him some peanuts!" Then I thought better of it and merely led Cam away, murmuring, "Gooble, gobble." The gawkers followed us with their eyes but said not a word.

When we learn that Bridget, Cam's gymnastics coach, also gives Saturday group lessons to developmentally disabled students, we decide to give one a try. As we pile into the car that day, I notice that Cam's hair is getting shaggy. "Hey, is it time to bring out the Flowbee?"

"Oh, Bunny!" Les breaks out laughing. "The Flowbee! What a silly thing!"

"Thank God we had it. Those haircuts were painful. He just couldn't wait."

When Cam was small, we'd tried to take him to a barber or stylist, but he was incapable of waiting for more than two minutes without throwing a fit, so we'd write his name on a list and go for a walk. Upon returning, we'd try to be brisk and matter-of-fact, but Cam would fidget, bounce, and emit ear-piercing wails. He was afraid that the haircut would hurt, and too often his perpetual motion made his fear come true. The barbers, God love 'em, were long-suffering, but there was only so much they could do.

Each haircut was worse than the last. Adults usually averted their eyes, but the kids were less tactful. One little boy, after observing Cam thrashing and screaming, turned to his mother and said, "That boy is bad, mommy!"

"He's just having a rough day," she said, trying not to smile.

We smiled back, but couldn't help but feel the kid was right: we were lousy parents raising a bad kid.

Cam had to get his hair cut somehow, so when he was five, Les bought a device called a Flowbee—electric clippers that you attach to a vacuum cleaner. I was skeptical: if anything was more likely to scare Cam than regular clippers, this was surely it. And when she hooked up the device, switched on the roaring machine and started toward Cam, he did flee in terror.

My wife was undeterred. She put the machine on her own head ("See, Cam, Mommy's cutting her hair!"), bribed him with snacks ("One more minute and you can have a cookie"), told him she'd cut only till we counted to ten. By the fourth haircut, he could make it to "six" before scurrying away. Most sessions ended with Les chasing Cam around the house with the vacuum cleaner, as if she were trying to suck him into the bag like a giant dust bunny.

With all of the chasing and bargaining, a haircut could take well over an hour. But at least we kept the mayhem within our own four walls.

Our chuckles die down as we pause at a stoplight. I take Les's hand. "Speaking of waiting, when was the last time we went to Salsa Grill?"

"A year or so ago, I guess. You think we should we try again?"

I make a raspberry sound: "Oh, no. 'It wouldn't be fair to the other customers.'"

For years we dined once a month at a nearby Tex-Mex place. The place was poorly run: five or six tables invariably sat empty, yet we always had to wait at least ten minutes while Cam dropped to the floor, writhed, hollered, clapped, and whined. Once we got a table, things usually smoothed out: we brought pretzels for Cam to munch, and he generally ate some of his grilled cheese sandwich and fries. Les and I wolfed down our meals and left as soon as we finished. It was far from a relaxed dining experience, but we thought it was good for all of us.

During one wait, Les asked to speak to the manager. A harried man in his early thirties met us in the foyer.

"This is Cameron. He has autism and gets very anxious and disruptive when he has to wait." She flashed her most ingratiating smile. "So we wondered if it would be possible for us to bypass the line and just walk in."

The manager gazed over her shoulder. "Well, I don't know. Everybody else has to wait their turn."

"True, but they're not disabled. They can see that he's different. I'll bet nobody would mind too much. If you could help us, we'd really appreciate it." She smiled again, more tightly.

The manager looked down at his shoes. "I'll have to ask my supervisors. And you can always have a seat in the bar; there's usually no wait there. But I tell you what. Why don't you call ahead next time? That way you'll be in the queue before you get here." He excused himself.

Les, her lips pressed together, turned to me. I knew that look too well. "Let's go."

But Cam didn't want to leave: we had come here to eat, and that's what he expected to do. As we groped for the door amid the crowd of people waiting, he screamed and threw himself to the floor. I lifted him up and, with one hand on his back and the other fending off his blows, hustled him toward the door. The line parted like the Red Sea, the children wide-eyed, the adults carefully looking somewhere else.

"I can't believe that little weenie!" Les said as we drove home. "Cam is disabled! You might as well ask a person in a wheelchair to get up and walk!"

"I suppose he's afraid somebody will complain. Everyone's ready to sue these days."

"Yeah, well, I might! It's illegal! I feel like calling their headquarters!"

Remembering how she'd once battled a hospital billing department for overcharging us, I didn't doubt it. Instead, the next time we planned to eat out, she called ahead, explained Cam's autism and asked if they could write our names down so we wouldn't have to wait.

The manager got on the phone. "We can put your name down, but if it's not the first name on the list when you get here, you'll still have to wait your turn."

"We've been coming to your restaurant for five years. I talked to you a few weeks ago about this, and you told me if we called ahead, we wouldn't have to wait. My son has severe autism. Surely you can make some accommodation." She didn't raise her voice; only her coldly precise enunciation revealed her anger.

"Well, it just wouldn't be fair to the other customers."

"You have a wheelchair ramp, don't you? This is no different!" Her voice had grown shrill.

"Give me your name, then. But I can't guarantee no wait."

"Forget it!" She slammed down the phone.

That was the last time we tried to eat there.

"That's one headache we don't need. But you did all you could, sweet-pea."

"No more eating out," Les sighs.

"Nope. No more movies either."

"Oh, God. I can't even bear to think of that."

I gingerly recall the painful episode. Four years earlier, the Disney animated feature *Oliver and Company* came to a local cinema. One of Cam's favorite sing-along videos featured tunes from the movie, so this seemed a great outing. He might get cranky, but he might be thrilled. We decided to give it a shot, selecting a Saturday matinee when we'd be less obtrusive.

We told him we were going to see a movie. "It's like a big TV, Cam. It'll be fun!"

Though he darted suspicious looks at us as we walked from the parking lot, Cam strode swiftly along, occasionally giving the single clap and crow-hop that means, "I'm excited!"

We bought popcorn and sodas, and for safety's sake sat in the last row on the aisle. Cam happily swigged his Coke, laughed, and bounced in his seat. When the lights went down, he turned to me. "Go to sweep?"

I squeezed his hand. "No, it's not bedtime, bud. We're gonna watch a movie! Remember, it's just like TV, only bigger!"

Satisfied for the time being, he slurped his drink and crunched popcorn as the trailers finished and the feature began. We thought he was behaving very well—only a little clapping and vocalizing—but the people directly in front of us didn't agree. A boy and a girl who looked about five or six kept turning around and whispering.

A few minutes into the movie Oliver, a stray kitten, gets introduced to city life by a wily pooch who sings, "Why should I worry? / Why should I care? /

I may not have a dime / But I've got street *savoir faire*." Cam couldn't believe his luck: he knew this song!

"Why should I worry!" he sang at the top of his voice, clapping loudly. "Oooh, looh, looh!"

The kids turned and gawked; their mom swivelled and gave us a stare that Garland-Thomson doesn't mention: the disapproving glower that means "You ill-bred morons!" She wasn't impressed with Cam's knowledge: we were ruining their movie-going experience.

Now would have been the time to explain to them matter-of-factly, "We're sorry he's so loud, but Cam has autism and can't help it. He'd really like to watch the movie too, so please ignore him." Instead we shrank down in our seats and tried to look inconspicuous.

Cam grew restless. At home he would have wandered into his room or bounced on the tramp. Denied those outlets, and unable, like Rain Man, to recite "Who's on First," he started to clap and belch emphatically. Now the whole row of faces to our right glared at us.

I wanted to stand up and announce, "Stop staring, you jerks! My son has as much right to be here as you do. More right, in fact, because this means more to him!" I wish I *had* done that instead of what we actually did: rise and exit the theater.

We walked rapidly, our eyes wide and blank. Cam, however, kept looking left and right at his parents. Why were we leaving?

"Could you believe those nasty looks?"

"Well, at least we got to see a few minutes of it. I think he enjoyed it."

Maybe. But he also retreated to his room and lay on his bed for the rest of the afternoon. Did he understand that his noises had spoiled things, or was he simply sad that we'd ended his fun? I fervently hoped that he hadn't grasped the message the others had sent: you're not one of us.

We too were dejected. We cursed autism but also cursed ourselves. We had chickened out, let embarrassment stand in the way of Cam's pleasure. We told ourselves we should have brazened our way through it instead of cravenly sacrificing Cam's enjoyment on the altar of civility.

This painful memory not only typified how Cam's autism had shrunk our world; it also crystallized our guilt for allowing it to shrink. We told ourselves to toughen up, and mostly we had.

At the gym that Saturday, Cam eagerly shows off his trampoline skills. Utterly fearless, he jumps far higher than anyone else.

We recognize many of the other boys, most of them also autistic. From behind the plate glass of the observation room, among the other parents chatting about soccer teams and piano lessons, I see the boys as others might. Some wave their fingers or vocalize; others walk with a lopsided gait; others carry plastic toddler toys. I proudly note that my son—a handsome boy with sleek brown hair and bright brown eyes—doesn't shuffle or gaze distractedly at the ceiling.

But then I detect the goofy, near-hysterical edge to his laugh. And when he drops to his knees, squeals, and shoves his fingers into his ears, my bubble of complacency bursts. The chasm between us and the scrubbed, perky moms and bored-looking pops yawns open. We need no chanting "freaks" to remind us we aren't part of their world.

I shrug. We'll just party with other autistic families. Yet when we join the other parents in the small gym next door, we're greeted with wary looks: they don't want a wild card upsetting their kids, whose coping abilities are fragile enough without him. They've heard about Cam and have told themselves, "At least my kid's not *that* bad." They barely acknowledge us.

As we drive off, Cam shouts, "Take a bath!" and grabs a handful of Les's hair. The lesson has upset him: it's a Saturday, other boys are there—not in the routine! But perhaps something else is on his mind. Agonizing questions rise up again: is he aware of his difference? Is he embarrassed by others' stares? Is he ashamed of being grouped with the "special" families?

At such times I actually hope his disability is severe enough to protect him from the arrows people shoot from their eyes. If he *does* know that others see him as a freak, victim, or spectacle, he might be quadruply wounded: not only by his disorder and its stigma, but also by the recognition of his difference and, worst of all, by his inability to compensate for it.

Of course, there's another possibility: he knows he's different but doesn't care. The truth is, I don't know.

Third base.

Certain people don't seem to notice Cam's behaviors. Such obliviousness may seem a blessing, but sometimes it adds to the torture. One morning in 2000, for instance, Cam and I stopped at a nearby café to get me an iced coffee and him a frozen treat. As we stood in line, I impatiently watched an obese woman and her meek husband dither over their order.

"I want a turkey and tomato sandwich, um, with, let's see. . . . Do you have mustard? What kind?"

"Dijon, ma'am," the clerk said, gesturing toward the sign listing available fixings.

"Oh, I don't like that kind. Well, how about tuna?"

"Sorry, we're out of tuna today."

"Oh. Well, then, the turkey and tomato with. . . . What kind of soft drinks do you have?"

"You have to order those at the other counter, ma'am."

"Oh, well, honey, why don't you order, while I go look."

While her hubby drawled out their order, Cam wandered to the card-and-party displays several feet away. Soon he was kneeling on the floor playing with a ribbon he'd pulled from a balloon. I wasn't sure what to do: if I fetched him I might lose our place in line, and if I made him stay with me I'd invite a calamity.

I trotted to him, snatched a plastic lei hanging nearby, traded it for the balloon, and returned to the line. Hubby was still placing his order.

Within seconds the lei was in tatters. I began to sweat. Stepping out of line again, I gathered up the strips and crammed them into my pocket. Meanwhile, the next person in line had moved forward. I returned to my place in front of her. She said nothing.

As the clerks slowly prepared the couple's orders, I drummed my fingers on the counter and sighed deeply. Heavy Gal shot a withering glance my way. Should I just leave? No: I'd still have to pay for the stupid plastic lei. Several minutes passed. Finally I ordered a cappuccino and frozen custard, then collected the bits of lei and heaped them on the check-out counter.

"Norma, how do I ring this up?" the clerk called to the manager, who was in no hurry to answer. Cam, still kneeling by the party display, clapped and made agitated "ooohhh" noises; any minute now he'd wet his pants. I dashed from the checkout and showed him his treat. "Come over here, buddy, and eat your ice cream."

I'm sure all of this took only seven or eight minutes, but it seemed as long as an afternoon at the Department of Motor Vehicles. I tried to keep my eyes blank and show no interest or excitement, but I could feel my face flushing and ears burning.

At last I joined Cam at the dining counter, where he gazed calmly out the window at the parking lot. Scornfully refusing the spoon I proffered, he insisted on eating the icy treat with a plastic fork he'd found.

Heavy Gal and Hubby sat at a booth directly behind us. I feigned insouciance while Cam gooble gobbled his custard. Then the tics began.

"Clap, clap, clap, clap, clap!" said his hands.

"Heeka deeka deeka deeka!" shouted his mouth.

"Hmmmm?!" He giggled and pushed his face next to mine.

I didn't look at Heavy and Hub.

Cam finished his treat. "Put it in the trash, dude," I said. He shoved the cup and fork into the garbage can, gave a hop, and headed barefoot for the door.

"Come back and put your sandals on."

As I buckled them on, he grumpily remarked, "Huh, huh, huh."

"Ready to go?" I asked.

"Ready," he replied. On the way out, he shouted for good measure, "Go!"
Just another day on Planet Autism.

A few days later, I found a "My Turn" column written by Robert Hughes in
an old issue of *Newsweek*. Hughes describes people's reactions to his autistic
son Walker, who also jams his fingers into his ears, skips, darts, and makes loud
noises. Hughes pinpoints what he calls "The Look": the concerned but smug
response folks register when they "diagnose" his son's autism. Walker, however,
seems to enjoy the attention: his actions say, "Here I am! Look at me!"

What struck me hardest was Hughes's conclusion: people's reactions derive
less from how the *son* acts than from how the *father* responds to him. If Dad
seems angry or ashamed or ambivalent, people pick up the cue and perceive
Walker as unruly, freakish, or pitiable. "Why shouldn't passersby stare at the
friendly son when the father's face is cloudy with conflict and questioning?" He
has learned to work on *his* look.

I put down the article and gazed up at Cam. Out of the corner of his eye, he
was staring right at me.

Chapter 15

In the Echo Chamber

... you speak at last
With a remote mime
Of something beyond patience,

Your gaping wordless proof
Of lunar distances
Travelled beyond love.
—Seamus Heaney, "Bye-Child"

"Bayto! Bayto!" Cameron is shouting. I pay attention, for he speaks so rarely. But what *is* he saying? "Bathtub?"

"You already had a bath, bud. It's time for bed."

That isn't it. He repeats "Bayto, bayto," for several minutes, each repetition more emphatic than the last. Finally he declares, "That hurt!" It's a rote phrase left over from one of our attempts to teach him not to hit people, and usually crops up completely out of context. This time he is trying to convey something specific, yet I can't for the life of me determine what it is. Leslie is usually better at deciphering his words, so I call her into Cam's bedroom.

"What was that all about?" I ask her afterward.

"Something hurt, I think," she answers, shaking her head.

"You think he really meant 'that hurt?'"

"Yeah. But I'm not positive."

After Cam falls asleep, we sit side by side on the sofa, recalling our long struggle to help him talk. We feel frozen in time, beset by scenes and sounds reverberating from years past.

Gloss

At ten months, Cam said "Hi," then added "raisin," "kitty cat," "dog," "cup," and a few other words. By age three he'd lost most of these and seemed utterly fogged in, confined to that looking-glass land where everyone spoke jabberwocky.

Gradually he began to understand a few simple, familiar words and phrases. But saying things was much tougher. Sometimes the more we tried, the worse things got. When he was about six, for example, we tried to teach him to frame requests with "I want": "I want to go outside," instead of just "outside." The goal was to build on single words until he could say full grammatical sentences. But "I want" flummoxed him, and after a few weeks of this training he developed a stammer. It was excruciating to watch his brown eyes blink and his lips tremble as he stuttered out, "Wah, wah, wah, wah." He'd stop, slap his chest and try again, only to be confounded by the same syllables. We'd give him as much time as he needed, but often he'd get so frustrated he'd just give up and howl or pinch his interlocutor.

Then one of our Lovaas therapists began placing her finger on Cam's chin to prevent tics; her tactic helped to defeat his stutter. For the entire summer of 1996, when he turned seven, Cam "wanted" everything in sight—food, the swing, rides, you name it. His confidence bloomed; his demeanor calmed.

When Diane Ellison heard that Cam was suddenly speaking in short, clear sentences, she was convinced we'd witnessed a miracle. "This is very unusual. Kids who are essentially nonverbal at five, like Cam was, almost never learn to talk." Our elation knew no bounds: our son had finally broken through into language!

But before long he began prefacing every request with "want to go," as in "Want to go cheese, yes." Both Diane and Cam's school speech pathologist assured us that "want to go" was a "verbal stim" (that is, a nonproductive utterance) and urged us to get rid of it. We tried: "Not 'want to go.' Say 'I want cheese.'" Cam: "Want to go I want cheese." The stutter returned; soon "want to go" went and nearly everything else went with it. Our efforts to improve his speech had only hampered it. We rued our misguided efforts: hope's budding made its wilting all the more devastating.

It's easy to imagine that a deep silence hangs over people with autism, but nothing could be further from the truth, at least in our case. Cam has always been a noisy, histrionic child. He speaks most volubly with his body, and over the years we've learned to interpret this language: the gleeful scissor-kicking jumps; the contented or angry rocking; the myriad wordless shouts; the fine gradations in a face that to the uninitiated seems blank; an entire lexicon of claps.

Cam's claps are his personal Morse code. A single clap after he has sung a line or done something he finds remarkable serves as an exclamation point: "How about that?!" A series of claps in front of his open mouth creates a booming effect that means "I'm getting mad," or "I wish I could tell you what I mean." Several loud claps and a grimace means "I'm anxious," or "I don't like what you told me" (for example, "stop splashing water outside of the tub"). And let's not forget those declarative rhythmic claps he favors in public places: "Cam is here!"

He also uses a few all-purpose words, such as "Coke" (which sometimes means "I want a Coke," but sometimes means "I want . . . something") or "car" ("I don't know where I want to go, but I want to get out of here"). And he never says plain old "no"; it's always "No, okay." Les and I inadvertently gave birth to this locution through conversations like this:

"Cam, do you want to go outside?"

"No."

"Okay."

The two words became a single thought. Those who don't know him are confused by the phrase: does he mean no or yes? To us it seems to encapsulate Cam's struggle with language: one word cancels the other.

Sometimes he gives forth a long stream of syllables that sound like gibberish but really aren't. Over the years we've learned to decrypt it.

Cam's Glossary

1. *"Loo, loo, loo,"* or *"loo-ee, loo-ee, ah loo-ee" (uttered in a low, even tone)* = "I'm really contented," or "I think you're cool," or "I'm pleased with myself." After a gymnastics lesson in 2000, Cam's coach told me that he seemed to like Louie, another boy in the group. "He kept saying, 'Louie, Louie, Louie.'" I didn't have the heart to tell her that he was just naming his own satisfaction.

2. *"Hooka, tooka, tooka"* = "This is really fun."

3. *"Hey, hooh, huuh"* = "I'm deep in thought."

4. *"Eeeh, geeta gee!"* = depending upon tone, anything from strong displeasure to panic.

5. *"Huh huh huh" (a fake laugh, followed by rocking)* = "Let's laugh together!"

6. *"Hmmmm?"* = "Are you noticing me?" (The proper response is "Hmmmm?" followed by a conspiratorial laugh.)

7. *"Cut-tik, cut-tik, cut-tik" (whispered)* = "I'm concentrating deeply."

I've often speculated that Cam's expressions are his version of Leslie's quirky wordplay. This is a woman who can't leave words alone. Thus "Watson" (her pet name for me) metamorphosed into "Wallace," then "Walmart" and "walnut," among others. Similarly, "to pee" evolved into "Peabo Bryson," and then into "bryson." A stupid person is not merely dim but "dimsky Korsakov" or a "nylonhead." A cold day isn't "chilly," it's "chili dog," or "Chilliwack" (fans of 1970s rock will recognize the allusion). How, we ask, could two such confirmed word lovers manage to produce a nearly wordless child?

Though Cam's sounds and multipurpose words do have meanings, they are blunt instruments—poor tools for expressing anything complex or precise. Hence, we've had to become detectives or telepaths, deducing our son's emotions, desires, and thoughts from his facial expressions, gestures, cryptic syllables. We've often failed at the guessing game, partly because his language is so rudimentary, partly because his thinking is so different from ours. At times we've felt like poor, beleaguered Alice, protesting to pugnacious Humpty Dumpty that "glory" doesn't mean, as he claims, "a nice knock-down argument."

"'When I use a word,' Humpty Dumpty said, in a rather scornful tone, 'it means just what I choose it to mean—neither more nor less.'"

Unlike Humpty, Cam can't enforce his definitions. Instead his language embodies the egg man's other major trait—fragility. Once Cam's language shattered, all of the teachers and all of the speech therapists couldn't put it together again.

Reverb

Starting when Cam was four, Les and I met yearly with his team of educators and therapists. Each year, we stressed the same points; we could have recorded the conversation when he was four and played it back when he was eleven: "We think the main focus should be on communication. If he can express his wishes, he won't have to resort to slapping, pinching, and biting." Every year, the team members nodded sagely and outlined a plan. And the next year, Cam had made little or no progress. We seemed to live in a gigantic echo chamber where our words bounced back at us year after year.

And so did Cam: for years, his spoken language consisted mostly of echolalia. The phenomenon is named for Echo, a nymph in Greek mythology charged with entertaining Queen Hera with lively talk. One day, when Hera was attempting to catch her husband, Zeus, frolicking with other nymphs, Echo's chattering distracted the queen from the task. She punished Echo by proclaiming that henceforth her speech would be limited to repeating someone else's last utterance. When Echo fell in love with the beautiful youth Narcissus, her echoing scared him off. Despondent, she retreated to mountain caves, and eventually faded away until nothing was left but her voice. Cam seemed to share her fate.

Many experts hold that echolalia isn't true language, that although typical children pass through an echolalic stage that functions as a bridge to true symbolic language, echoing lacks the originality, spontaneity, and give-and-take of real conversation. Special educator Adriana Schuler and speech pathologist Barry M. Prizant argue that when an autistic person quotes a TV show or commercial—as many love to do—he or she is using only lower brain structures; no real language is being spoken. Famed neurologist Oliver Sacks even claims that autistic echolalia is "purely automatic" and "carries no emotion, no intentionality."

Cam's echolalia did often sound like mechanical parroting. If, for example, we asked him, "Do you want a banana or an orange?" he would probably say "orange"; but if we reversed the order, he'd say "banana." He couldn't seem to remember that we'd offered two choices. Even when we coached him, his "improved" responses were often just redoubled echoes: "Do you want bread?" "Bread." "Don't repeat; say 'yes.'" "Yes." "Do you want bread?" "Bread, yes."

But other researchers have shown that echolalia serves a variety of linguistic functions, and autistic authors such as Jasmine O'Neill and Donna Williams write that their childhood echolalia gave them time to process others' words and a way to join conversations. In any case, our own experiences have proven Sacks's hypothesis wrong, or at least incomplete. For example, in the bread exchange, Cam isn't just echoing; he's also assenting. Schuler and Prizant cite cases of "situation-association," in which people use echolalia to comment on their surroundings by linking current activities with previous events or occasions. Sometimes the scripts have a metonymic relationship with the circumstances. Thus when Cam, at four, wanted to end a speech therapy session, he used a memorized script, "Take your shoes off," by which he meant "Put your shoes on"—that is, "let's get ready to go home."

Cam still uses phrases he learned from those old toddler books or kids' songs to express himself. Hence, when he looks at Les or me and says, "Guess what, Max?" we are to respond with "What?"—the next sentence in the book *Max's Christmas*, which he memorized at age two—and then we *must* recite the entire book. These questions and answers may not be "true" conversation, but they involve give and take, shared attention and associations. They are his way of asking for help or intimacy. (Others can misinterpret these phrases. Once Cam's teacher called home, extremely excited that he'd said, "What happened? Be calm," and "Who are you talking to?" She had no idea that these were phrases [mis]quoted from *Max's Christmas*.)

Sometimes an echo's meaning is quite clear. One morning, for example, he bounded into our room, crawled into our bed, and led us through *Barney*'s theme song: "*I love you, you love me / We're a happy family. . . .*" He knew exactly what he meant and so did we. I've always hated that song, but when Cam sang it, the saccharine sentiment carried a redeeming poignancy.

Such incidents inspire wonder at his capacity to comment on his world, to compensate for his disability by selecting the right script. And once in a while, his ritualized monologues become less cryptic as he composes an idiosyncratic "mash-up" that mixes snatches of songs, words, and near-words in a strange and beautiful poetry: "Heeka-deeka duh, ah loo, ah loo, ah yuh you, hoppeen on one foot, huh-huh." It's as though he has traveled to some distant place and is reporting what he's seen there. Who could doubt that these strategies, which Paul Collins likens to a magpie building its nest from stray flotsam, display creativity and intelligence?

Yet Cam's inability to generate novel phrases remains deeply debilitating. Sometimes, for instance, the rote scripts interfere with his meaning. Let's say he wants to go for a ride, and we ask him to use proper words.

"Cam, what do you want?"

"Car."

"Can you say 'I want to go in the car?'"

"Car, yes."

"I want."

"Want."

"To go."

"Go."

"In the . . ."

"Bed."

Why does he say "bed" when he means car? Because "in the" precedes "bed" in the memorized phrase "sleep in the bed." He seems to forget the original request once the sentence is broken into parts, and instead of recalling that in this context the phrase ends with "car," he lets the script "in the bed" usurp it. Yet he knows full well that "bed" is the wrong answer. So after saying "bed," he'll growl or clap angrily, as if to say, "Damn it, I don't know why I said that, because it isn't what I meant."

Sentences are thin-shelled eggs; once broken, they can't be reassembled.

We neuro-typical people flip through our mental rolodex until we find the mot juste—the appropriate word with the right nuances. Usually we retrieve at least an approximation. But even when Cam has used a particular word many times, he still must hunt laboriously for it like someone looking for pictures in a dark, crowded attic. He'll stare into your eyes and scan your face intently. You gaze back at him, trying to *will* the words into his mind. He grabs the closest approximation—a garbled word, a metonym—but there may be no picture for what he wants to say. How, for example, can his concrete mind convey something like, "I'm anxious about entering this noisy, unfamiliar building?" Shouting "Coke!" won't really do the job.

When Cam was about nine, we started using assistive technology devices. The first was an Easy Talk machine (a console of large buttons with pictures pasted on them; you push the button and it says a recorded phrase). We replaced that with the Language Master. It was eerie to hear my voice trying to make routine outings— "go to Burger King"—sound like glorious escapades. Eerier was the feeling that the machine had snatched Cam's lost words from the ether to give them fleeting expression.

The machine said what he couldn't and said it clearly every time. But we could never create enough cards for all the possible situations in his life: the machine could not say, "I feel sick," or "I'm afraid," or "That sound hurts my ears."

Noted autistic author Temple Grandin writes that she thinks not in words but in pictures. Does Cam? Is his head filled with a slide show of captionless illustrations? If so, does he maintain that voice in his head that comments on his activities, makes long- and short-term plans, tells him what to do next? Sacks theorizes that many autists can't connect individual experiences into a continuous narrative and thus exist in a pure present of "vivid, isolated moments, unconnected with each other or with [themselves]." Anyone living in such a "pure present" would seem to lack the self-awareness we identify with true human consciousness.

Our son *has* sometimes behaved as if he lived in a pure present, failing to remember an activity from one day to the next or not recognizing people he's known for years. But sometimes he says something so appropriate you know he must tell his own story.

For instance, when he was about five we drove from Baltimore to Atlantic City so I could take the test to become a *Jeopardy!* contestant. The long day tapped out Cam's shallow reserves of patience. As we wearily rode the elevator back to the parking lot, two grizzled gents, reeking of smoke and stale liquor, boarded the car with us. This was the final indignity: as soon as the door thumped shut Cam started shrieking. Then, suddenly, he stopped and shouted, with perfect clarity, "I need to go crazy!"

One of the casino habitués nodded sagely and said, "We feel the same way, kid."

Cam had made perfect sense: this elevator is too small, I don't know these people, and I want to scream! Such moments prove that he *does* narrate his life and even has some understanding of his condition. They also remind us how often he reaches for words but comes up empty. And they make me wonder: does he think fluently in words but stumble only when trying to say them?

Other linguistic eccentricities invite further speculation. For example, Cam often uses "I" for "you" and "he" for "I." Since nobody has ever called him "I," he figures—with sound autistic logic—that he is "he." But he's not sure. So he takes a middle ground, employing a pronoun that combines "he" and "I": "Ee take a baff."

If a person has trouble using "I," you have to wonder if he thinks of himself *as* an "I." Perhaps Cam lives at a distance from himself, responding to his own acts with bewilderment, as if they've issued from some other "he"—maybe the other person he calls into being when he watches his fingers create shadows. On the other hand, perhaps the problem is that he *can't* imagine himself as another person might see him. Such a "theory of mind" dysfunction (the notion that autistic people don't understand others' thoughts) would suggest that Cam's problem is not that he's too distant from himself, but that he can't distance himself from his own thoughts and actions, can never see outside his own obsessions, never breach the walls of his echo chamber.

Because our son was so aloof and so seldom talked, we fell into the habit of treating him as if he couldn't hear. When we was very young and nothing seemed to penetrate his cocoon, he might as well have been deaf. In later years, however, he occasionally showed us quite plainly that he understood our words. One day I was talking with our head therapist about how hard it was for Cam to think of the right words and started recounting the history of his language problems. After a couple of minutes, he put his head on her shoulder, then approached me, growling and gnawing fiercely on his rubber chew toy.

The truth dawned on me: "I think he wants us to stop talking about him," I said. "I think it bothers him." She nodded: first he seemed to want sympathy, then had acted embarrassed, and finally irritated. I realized with chagrin that we'd been treating him like an infant or pet. Our life might have been easier if he were: at least then we could reliably estimate his cognitive abilities.

One morning, after Les told Cam—then aged eleven—that he couldn't go outside until after breakfast, he launched into one of his wordless monologues, concluding with a phrase that sounded like, "That's annoying."

"Did you hear that?" Leslie said to me.

"I did. Is that even possible?"

We shook our heads, wondering all over again if normal language lay somewhere in his brain, misfiled and unavailable. When those spotlights of comprehension shine through the fog of the disorder, you no longer trust your judgment. The worst such moments—such as that fateful evening when he shouted "trapped!"—only make his condition more agonizing for all of us. In the wake of such utterances, our hard-won accommodation to reality is, like Humpty's shell, shattered all over again.

The night Cam shouts "Bayto!," I have a dream I've had before. I'm falsely accused of some vague crime. Though innocent, when I try to defend myself in court, I am tongue-tied: I literally cannot open my mouth. I wake in a cold sweat and stumble into the bathroom to wipe my face. I think about how, in barbaric societies, traitors and informers get their tongues cut out. As I look in the mirror, it strikes me that my nightmare is my son's waking life. Cam has never done anything wrong, yet he has spent his life, in effect, tongueless. A wave of nausea courses through me. I gag. Eventually I push down the sickness, but there is no more sleep that night.

The next morning Les calls me into Cam's room. "Bunny, look at this." She points to Cam's big toe: it is bruised and blue, the cuticle crusted with dried blood.

"Oh my God," I say. "'Big toe!' That's what he was trying to tell us last night! How stupid am I? I thought he was saying 'bathtub.'"

I had dismissed his words as echolalia. His meaning now seems obvious: his toe was throbbing, but he couldn't make his dense parents understand.

That hurt.

Thinking again of the hardships my son faces every day, I am briefly overcome by sadness. But then I realize that, in trying to communicate despite his disability, in seeking to escape from his echo chamber, Cam displays "something beyond patience": something like heroism. He has never given up trying to talk. How, then, can we ever stop listening?

Part Three

Emergenc(i)es

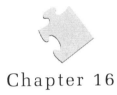

Chapter 16

Fighting Words

What's gone
is common happiness
plain bread we could eat
with the old apple of knowledge
—Denise Levertov, "Prisoners"

The Cuckoo in the Nest

A few days after summer school began in 2000, Cam jumped out of the car, ran to the road's edge, and began picking branches from our three dogwoods.

"Not off the trees, Cam. You know the rules. Now you have to go in the house."

As we stepped inside he swung from his heels and smacked me right in the testicles.

"Yow! That hurts!" I bellowed, grabbing him by the shoulders. "Why are you doing that?!" Remembering the guilt I'd felt the week before camp when I thought I'd bruised him, I took a deep breath, carefully maneuvered him into the living room and closed the kitchen door.

Cam wailed. Why was Daddy so mad? A few minutes later I sat down beside him. He clutched my hand and sobbed, "I sowwy, I sowwy."

"Cam, you can't hit people. It makes them very mad. And it hurts. You hurt Daddy!"

"Uh-uh, uh-uh, uh-uh." He rocked and chewed on his shirt.

"Are the big boys at school scaring you? You'll get to used to it, son. They'll be your friends pretty soon," I said. He looked directly into my eyes; I saw a flicker of comprehension.

The reason for this outburst was no mystery: without warning us, the school had moved Cam to a new classroom with a new teacher and new peers—which didn't include Andrew, his first and only friend. He'd been anxious ever since.

On the evening of the first day, a Wednesday, he couldn't get to sleep. I'd told him gently that he was getting to be a big guy and needed to do new things. Les gave him a hug, adding, "Miss Tracy said you were *so* smart. You're moving up because you're doing so well!"

He soon snuggled down and fell asleep. All things considered, he'd handled the first day pretty well. But Cam often has a delayed reaction to trauma. I wrote in my journal, "The real test will come around next Monday."

It didn't even take that long. On Saturday, Cam slapped Leslie and tried to bite me when he had to wait two minutes for a peanut butter sandwich. He roamed and rampaged the rest of the afternoon. Monday brought the outburst I described above.

Cam's just-completed stay at Camp Wonder had given us time to reflect, recharge our batteries, and regain perspective. Only a week later, those bright days already seemed long ago.

A war began to consume our household. The primary front was the battle between Cam and me. Leslie tried to mediate, but her presence sparked further hostilities, as her motherly instincts struggled against her wifely loyalty. Les and I waged a separate war over our individual moments of privacy, and as the summer passed, the already slender threads of our patience and endurance frayed even further.

I truly believed I was handling things well—further testimony to my superhuman powers of denial. But two incidents within twenty-four hours brought the truth home to me.

At 5:30 p.m. on July 13—ten days after camp—I ordered pizza for Cam and myself. By 6, Cam was loudly insisting, "I want a Coke."

I explained that we had to wait for the pizza man and could get a Coke afterward. No use: the obsession had gripped him. For the next several minutes, he ran through his entire menu of phrases, each more vehement than the last. He ended with: "Mommy! Seben [7–11]. Go!"

Where was the pizza man? And where was Leslie?

I called the pizza parlor. "He should be on his way," the young man told me.

"Well, he'd better be. If he's not here by 6:25 we're leaving," I warned. "I've got a kid here who's freaking out!"

Hoping to distract Cam, I let him go outside. But when he realized the car door was locked, he wrenched at my shirt and screamed, "Car, car!"

"Listen, buddy, we just have to wait a couple of minutes for the pizza and then we can go." Too late: he snapped at my hand and tried to head-butt me. To prevent a front-yard wrestling match, I pushed him back into the house. He stomped into the living room, threw himself down on the couch, and bounced frantically, shouting at the top of his voice.

"Car! Coke! Coke! In the car? In the car!"

At last the pizza arrived. But Cam was far too agitated to eat. I gobbled two slices while he roared "Coke!" in my ear. At last we drove to Burger King, and by the time we returned home, he was singing happily. I knew I should have taken him for a Coke immediately, pizza be damned. I didn't understand my own behavior: I seemed to be setting up confrontations. It seemed as if I *wanted* to infuriate my son, *wanted* to punish him. But why?

The next morning Cam woke up extra early and crawled into bed with me. As we lay there giggling and cuddling, I wondered how I could have been angry at the little otter. I was soon reminded: even that slight variation in his routine disturbed him. Since he'd been awake longer than usual, he assumed that the bus was late or that he wasn't going to school that day, and when Leslie opened the door to leave, he slipped outside, shouted "Coke!" and ran down the driveway to the street where the car was parked.

I stood in the driveway and shouted, "Cam, come on back up here. We can't get a Coke because the bus will be here in a few minutes. Today is Friday and you're going to school. Don't you want to go to school?"

"Uhmer ona ita ita school bus."

I took a chance. "Okay, bud, let's go up the hill and wait for the bus." Cam trudged reluctantly beside me up the slope to the corner. But when we reached the crest and he saw no bus, he grabbed the neck of my shirt and pulled down hard, then grabbed a handful of chest hair and yanked.

"Back to the house. Now!"

Easy to say, not easy to do: he wouldn't budge. We stood in the middle of the suburban street, a father and son locked face to face in stalemated combat. With Cam's fingers still knotted in my shirt and hair, I start walking him backward down the hill. He pulled harder; I slipped out of my shirt. The scratches on my arms and chest pulsing red in the morning light, I slowly backed him down the hill to our yard. During this grappling dance, he landed several blows to my arms, shoulders, and chest.

Then he smacked me hard on the side of the head. Instinctively I snatched his hair and jerked his head back. Sure, I was trying to protect myself, but I was also royally pissed at this monstrous child who wouldn't stop attacking me.

At last I wrestled my son into the house. Bawling, his mouth contorted, his arms waving futilely, he approached me—as if to give me a hug—still growling under his breath. For once I had a pretty good idea of what he was feeling because I felt the same way: angry, frustrated, sad. But I couldn't even feel sorry for him; I could feel only my own rage and helplessness.

I gazed at the ceiling, forced myself to breathe deeply, then said as quietly as I could, "Buddy, the bus is on the way. Please calm down." He stalked around the living room clapping, his shirt stuffed into his mouth.

A minute or two later, the bus arrived, right on time. Why couldn't it have been early just this once?

I couldn't shake off the incident. For the rest of the day, I kept remembering the agony and confusion on Cam's face as he'd tried to hug me. My son was drowning, and he was taking us down with him. I huddled on the couch, staring glumly at the floor. "Our lives are shit," I thought. I remembered the pediatrician's words when we'd told him that Cam had PDD: "this isn't a death sentence." He was right: it's a life sentence.

I called Les and recounted the incident, trying to put up a brave front. "Cam's gone now, and I'm fine. I'll call Karen Nestor [the school behavior specialist] and ask her advice." Even though I'd told her—pretty convincingly, I thought—to stay at work, she insisted on coming home immediately. As I hung up, tears rose to my eyes. I was starting to hate my own child. Worse: I was beginning to fear him. What would happen in a couple more years, when he was my size?

Les suggested that I start seeing a shrink. I scoffed: I had no faith in psychiatrists. "We'll work through this somehow," I said. But I didn't believe myself.

Instead, I did what I always do when faced with a problem—looked for a book about it. I reread *Children with Autism*. What I found was not reassuring: the book said that many autistic kids have a tough time during adolescence. Some start having seizures; most lack the social skills and language to adjust to the ordinary problems of puberty. "Jesus," I thought, "this could get worse?"

A few days later I perused Anne Alvarez and Susan Reid's anthology, *Autism and Personality*. In her essay, Reid compares living with an autistic child to "having a cuckoo in the nest: the autistic child takes more and more of the family resources, but is unable to give anything much back." Her case study draws a chilling picture of desperate, beleaguered parents afraid to leave their house, totally cut off from friends and relatives. The imprisoned family, she writes, embodies "the imprisonment of the child within the autistic condition."

I swallowed hard: that was us, all right.

In another essay, Trudy Klauber analyzes parents' reactions to "the loss of the expected 'normal' child" and to "the constant daily strain of living with bizarre, avoidant, strange or totally uncommunicative behavior." Some family members, she writes, show signs of post-traumatic stress disorder; they resist treatment or are hostile to professionals. Certain parents, she continues, may perceive their child as "an alien . . . for whom they are responsible and whom they consciously accept and unconsciously may resent or sometimes hate."

I winced. I resisted treatment. I was always comparing Cam to an alien. And hadn't I felt something like hatred for him just days earlier?

Dragons

Knowing that other parents shared my experiences made me feel a little less alone. But the books didn't tell me what to do about any of it. A few days later I unexpectedly came across more helpful advice in a passage from the great German poet Rainer Maria Rilke's *Letters to a Young Poet*. "The only courage . . . demanded of us," he writes, "[is] courage for the most extraordinary, the most singular, and the most inexplicable [events] that we may encounter. . . . Perhaps all the dragons of our lives are princesses who are only waiting to see us once beautiful and brave. Perhaps everything terrible is in its deepest being something helpless that wants help from us."

I gazed up at the double-ring quilt on our living room wall; it suddenly looked like a suit of chain mail. My son was the terrible, helpless being, and I was the one who had to help him. I put down the magazine with renewed determination: I would not give in to despair no matter how much the dragon roared or how hot the cave became.

My vow wasn't tested right away. In fact, the next morning Cam wanted to play on the bed with me. He pulled me down onto the mattress and squealed in delight as I tickled him. He sniffed my head and feet, and we sang, "If you're happy and you know it." Yet that day his school report listed forty-four aggressive incidents.

The test came a couple of weeks later, when he again started perseverating on Coke during a drive. As we waited in the McDonald's drive-through, he thrust his foot forward and kicked my right shoulder repeatedly. I tried to immobilize his foot by leaning on it, but that only made him angrier.

"Do you want a Coke?"

"Coke."

"Then put your foot down."

He pulled it away, but five seconds later stuck it back up in my face. I elbowed it out of the way. He screwed his face into a grimace, screamed, and threw himself back on the seat.

I closed my eyes and thought of dragons and princesses.

After we bought the Coke, I pulled into the parking lot. "Now we're going to drive home. But we're not going anywhere unless you keep your foot back. IF you want this Coke, you have to sit up like a good boy."

He sat up straight. But as soon as I handed him the drink, he shoved his foot at me again. I stopped the car and got out.

"Put your foot back," I said. He pulled it back. I got back into the car. He kicked my shoulder. I got out again. A woman walking to her car stopped and stared. Cam and I performed this ridiculous minuet for another five minutes. When he finally tired of it, I drove home, fuming all the way: "What's with that damn foot, anyway? Does he want to stop? Go? Or is he just trying to get my attention?"

Sticking to my vow wasn't going to be easy.

A few days later, Cam hollered for a Coke and a banana, then kicked me repeatedly all the way to his gymnastics lesson. At the gym, the coach invited him to sit on a swing. Two other boys about Cam's age sat nearby: one sucked his thumb; another whined and threw himself down on the mat.

"M-M-M-ooo. M-m-m-eee," the boy pleaded. "Mommy, mommy, mommy, mommy."

"Mommy isn't here. She wants you to play here and have fun," the coach answered.

The boy cried louder. "Daddy, daddy, daddy, daddy," he said.

"Daddy's at work."

The whine became a shriek. The boy bounded around the room and flung himself to the mat again. Cam swung placidly at the far side of the room.

I suddenly realized that Cam's behaviors were like the other boy's whining, and for a moment saw our relationship objectively: an anxious child trying to share his fears with his unbending father. He hadn't wanted a Coke or a banana; he'd just wanted my reassurance. But all I could offer were rules and cold commands—fighting words.

The war escalated a few evenings later, when Cam asked for oatmeal at 10 p.m. and Les refused to give him any. He thrashed and howled for fifteen minutes. She went to comfort him. When I heard her cry out, I burst into Cam's room to find her holding her arm and grimacing. He had bitten her again.

"Cameron!" I said menacingly, stalking toward him. Imagine my shock when Leslie set herself between us and assumed a boxer's stance.

"Mark, move away. You're not going to yank him out of bed."

"*You* get out of the way!"

"You're out of control! I'm not moving!" Her hands were raised as if to fend off blows.

"*Get out of the way!*" I started to push her aside, then thought better of it. "What the fuck are you doing, Leslie? I'm not going to hurt him, for God's sake."

She remained in a crouch, palms spread in front of her, defending her child.

"Okay. Have it your way. Next time he can take your whole arm off for all I care." I stomped out and slammed the door.

Later the argument resumed. "What did you think I was going to do? Jesus, Les, I was trying to protect you."

"No, you weren't, you were going to take your anger out on him!"

"Well, he's the one who slaps, pinches, and bites, isn't he? Anyway, you know damn well I'm not going to hurt him. The worst I've ever done is slap his bottom," I said, conveniently forgetting the time I'd pulled his hair and the time I'd shaken his shoulders.

"Mark, you need to look at yourself. You want to hurt him, and I'm not going to let that happen."

"That's ridiculous. What is wrong with you?" I rose. "I'm not talking about this anymore."

I told myself I should have known better than to come between a mother bear and her cub. Les needed to blame somebody and I was handy. But as I lay in bed that night, I wondered if she was right. Did I want to punish Cam? Was I inciting tantrums so I could vent my anger at him?

The next morning I returned to Klauber's essay and read, "The child . . . may, in his silence, easily represent hated aspects of his parents' selves or their internal parental figures." It suddenly struck me that living with Cam was not so different from living with my father, an emotionally volatile person with a drinking problem. Was our warfare an echo of past father-son encounters? Was I provoking Cam so I could somehow pay back my dad? Was the dragon I wanted to slay Cam's autism or my father? Or was it myself? Had Cam become a symbol of my helplessness against the autism monster?

The next night Les had to work late. Cam and I got Chinese take-out that included what Les calls "rice packs"—those little boxes of rice and soy sauce. Afterward, he and I played hide-and-seek. At 10:30 I checked on him. He looked up drowsily as I stood over him, then raised his right arm, crooked it around my shoulders, and pulled me toward his body. I hugged him and spoke softly into his ear.

"Daddy's here, and everything's all right. You're Daddy's good boy. I love you. Now go to sleep, son."

He gave a sleepy smile and a look that said, "That's my dad!"

A block formed in my throat: the dragon had vanished, and a prince had taken its place.

Reckoning

As the dreadful summer of 2000 drew to a close, I felt I'd purged my anger. Here's what I wrote in my journal that September:

I've finally accepted Cam for what he is. That's what this summer has taught me. Yet I'm still plagued by the fear of selling him short. So I'm pulled two ways: if I don't accept his limitations, his otherness, I'll forever torture him and myself with unfair expectations. But if I give up, I might douse the one spark that could light his fire. It's hard to know which is worse.

I've learned other lessons this summer: that Cam craves independence; that he has the same needs and desires as other kids—to have friends; to feel important, successful, and loved; to try new things; to tease, challenge, test. All these limitations and eccentricities make him human—only more so. But it's still hard to love the human while hating the monster that turns him into a dynamo of tics, obsessions, anxieties, and frustrations.

The greatest lesson, though, has been seeing my own inner war refracted in his daily struggles.

I felt positive enough about our life that, when asked to give an address on "the life of the mind" in October, I presented Cam's autism as an opportunity to understand a unique human mind—as a gift, not a curse.

That November we decided to give Saturday group gymnastics lessons one more try. We were picking our way through the foyer jammed with boisterous kids and chattering parents when Cam darted toward the soda vending machine.

"No, buddy," I said. "We're going to the gym. No Coke right now."

We'd covered about five steps in the other direction when Cam snatched the hair of a four-year-old girl. Her eyes bulged; she shrieked in terror. Her mother shouted, "Stop! Stop! Oh, no!" Cam's face registered nothing.

A disturbing tableau formed in the crowded lobby: a father holding his son, trying to dislodge the boy's hands from the hair of a tiny, howling girl; her mother helplessly wringing her hands and repeating, "It's okay, honey, it's okay"; the boy's mother crouching beside him and saying gently, "Buddy, calm down. Calm down now, sweetie."

The father, however, was bellowing. "Cam, let go!"

"Mark, you're making it worse. Get away! Get away!" Les half-shouted through gritted teeth. The effort of restraining her fury had turned her face bright red.

"I'm trying to free his hands!"

"Let go!" she yelled again. Quietly, she said to Cam, "Let go now, sweetie. Give Mommy your hand."

Feeling that my head was about to explode, I flung my hands up and drew back.

At last Cam released his hold and fell to his knees. "Eeeh, eeeh, eeeh!" he screeched, pounding on the carpeted floor.

I jerked him roughly to his feet and pushed/pulled him out the door toward the car. The asphalt parking lot packed with vans, the nearby trees—it all seemed unreal, a phony painted backdrop for the violent family drama unfolding in front of it.

Cam collapsed again. I shouted, "Cameron, you pulled that girl's hair! That hurt her!" I wrestled him to a sitting position. "Bad! Bad! Bad!" He knocked my glasses off.

Leslie came running up behind us and opened the car door. She too was screaming—at me. "Mark! Let him up! You're over the top! Leave him alone!"

At last Cam stood up and trotted to the car. Les entered the driver's side. I stood on the pavement panting. I felt dazed; I couldn't move. At last I retrieved my glasses and fell into the passenger's seat.

"Jesus Christ!" I said, shaking my head.

Leslie was furious. "You are out of your mind! What is wrong with you!?"

"He was pulling the girl's hair. What was I supposed to do?"

"You asshole! You wanted to hurt him!" She turned to me, glasses askew, face purplish. "If you don't get professional help, I'm leaving you!"

Stunned, I stared at the floor.

"You've been angry at him for years. You need to find somebody to help you handle it. We can't go on like this! You are losing it!"

We sustained a clenched silence on the drive home and resumed the argument later. Les got to the point: "I'm very, very worried that you're going to injure him. You know you'll never forgive yourself if that happens. And I won't forgive you either." She pinned me to the couch with a glare.

I closed my eyes and recalled the summer of public outbursts and family fights. The few happy moments seemed like distant pinpoints of light in a cold, dark sky. I opened my eyes and looked at my hands. Autism was destroying our family. Not only was I was powerless to stop it, but I seemed to be abetting it. And now my wife—the only other reliable soul on our tiny craft—was turning against me too. I knew she was right. But I had no idea what to do.

A hopeless silence reigned for several minutes. Then I called on a lifelong habit: use logic. Maybe reason would prevail where emotion failed; maybe it could shed some light on our darkness. I reminded her that, through the years of madness, we had not only maintained careers but thrived professionally: she'd risen to the director level in her agency; I'd published books, won awards, made full professor.

"Yeah, but at what cost?" she asked. "I should never have gone back to work. I could have given all my time to Cam. We'd all be better off."

"You think so?" I recalled the dispirited mother at the parents' meeting in June. "Remember Martha? If you'd stayed home with Cam, you'd be just like her: a zombie, a rag doll. I would have withdrawn completely, and you'd hate me for it."

"Maybe so. But Wallace, you have an anger problem. Admit it."

I crossed my arms. "I don't have an anger problem. I have an autism problem." I rose from the couch. "And so do you."

"Mark, you are lying to yourself. I want you to get help before somebody gets hurt. I've asked you and asked you and asked you! Why won't you do it?" She was shouting again.

I looked out the window at a man walking his dog. Another long silence ensued. Then I gazed at my wife, the circles under her eyes betraying her bone-deep weariness. "Okay. I'll see a shrink. As long as you go with me."

Things had bottomed out: I had nothing to lose by asking for help.

Chapter 17

May Day!

In a dark time, the eye begins to see.
—Theodore Roethke

I was wrong. The worst was yet to come.

On Thursday, May 3, 2001, as I sat at our kitchen table, preparing for the yearly meeting to discuss Cameron's IEP, some lines from Emily Dickinson came to mind:

> Pain—has an Element of Blank—
> It cannot recollect
> When it begun—or if there was
> A time when it was not.

The pain of the past two months seemed to stretch backward to infinity; as I recalled them, the blank was filled by confusion, sadness, and fear. The upcoming meeting, the culmination of these months, would commit us to a decision that would change our lives forever.

Eruptions

To be in such a sorry state seemed especially cruel because the traumatic year 2000 ended with our best Christmas ever. For once we found a gift that Cam actually loved—an enormous stuffed St. Bernard we named Bernie. Cam himself picked Bernie from a pile of stuffed animals at F. A. O. Schwarz, and spent a good part of Christmas Day lying on the critter. He'd slept with Bernie every night since. Though just as faithful as a real dog, Bernie also offered a distinct advantage: he'd never chase or bite.

Over the rest of the winter, Cam went on field trips and made some academic progress. The crisis seemed to blow over, and we let the question of family therapy lapse. Then one day in early March, as Cam performed his after-school ritual of branch stripping, I noticed that his lips and the little furrow under his nose were twitching every few seconds. He'd licked his lips so much that a red ring had formed around them.

The next day his tics seemed more pronounced, so I forced myself to look up the side effects of Risperdal in the accompanying brochure. With mounting unease, I scanned the description of tardive dyskinesia: "a neurological syndrome characterized by repeated, involuntary jaw or lip movements." If you saw such movements you should contact your doctor immediately: they could become permanent. I gazed out at the maple trees swaying in the brisk March wind. I felt sick to my stomach.

The next morning I called Dr. Cohen. "Cam is making odd movements with his lips and mouth. The little cleft between the lips and nose—what's that called?"

"The filtrum?"

"It's twitching. And he's licking his lips constantly."

"Uh-hmm." He sounded bored. "And how often are these movements occurring?"

"Every minute or two, maybe more. We're worried. Could this be tardive dyskinesia?"

"Well, it is possible, but not likely."

"Yeah, we're probably overreacting. But could I come in tomorrow and show you what I mean?"

The next morning he observed Cam, and within two minutes concluded that the movements were "consistent with tardive dyskinesia." The nose twitching, he informed me, is called "rabbit syndrome" or "rabbiting"; though not serious, it's considered a "drug-emergent dyskinesia." He didn't hide his surprise: Risperdal was supposed to have an extremely low rate of such side effects. He didn't tell me why he hadn't noticed them until I'd brought them to his attention. But he recommended lowering Cam's dosage by 20 percent and watching him for a week.

A rough week ensued: Cam was irritable, anxious, aggressive. The dilemma was clear: if we took Cam off Risperdal, his aggression would explode; if we kept him on it, he might develop permanent tics and tremors.

Instead Cohen put Cam on Seroquel, a new, supposedly similar medication. Cam's moods only became more volcanic: if he had to wait thirty seconds for a snack, he'd slap Les or pull her hair; if we asked him to put his dish in the sink, he'd pinch the nearest hand; if I told him to move from the front yard to the back, he'd grab my shirt, gouge my hand, or threaten to bite.

We stopped taking him out of the house. We tiptoed around to avoid upsetting him. Monitoring him consumed every waking moment, and when he finally went to bed, Les and I huddled together, dazed and exhausted, on the sofa.

After a week, I reported to Dr. Cohen.

"That sounds unpleasant. It seems as if the Seroquel is not working."

"I'll say. It's making him worse." It took all of my strength not to scream, "For God's sake, man, *do something!*"

But we didn't know whether Cam's behaviors were caused by the Seroquel or by the reduction of Risperdal. To limit the variables, the doctor recommended we take him off all medications.

After three years, Cameron was suddenly med-free.

The next week was nightmarish. Even when Cam's aggression had spiked during 2000, we'd usually been able to discern *some* reason for his outbursts. But now his moods swung violently without warning or motive: one minute he was giggling, singing loudly, begging to be tickled, and the next minute he was furiously pinching, scratching, or slapping someone. In the space of seconds, he switched from roaring like a wounded lion to infantile whining for his mommy. Several times a day he burst into tears.

The worst part wasn't the aggression; it was what we had to do to protect ourselves. At 5' 3" and 100 pounds, Cam was becoming terribly hard to handle during a meltdown: it was almost impossible to move him to his room or protect yourself from his butting, biting, and scratching. Soon someone was going to get seriously hurt.

We tried to read his mind, which in some ways was not hard. Obviously he was wondering, "What are these things I'm feeling?" His emotions had been muzzled for so long that he no longer recognized them in all their natural power. The imp that Risperdal had kept bound up—the one that drove him to cram anxious fingers into his ears, went wild if a desire was thwarted, deflected his energy into compulsions—that creature had been sprung from its cell.

In earlier years, I used to gain solace by envisioning Cam without autism, picturing our athletic son playing baseball, our handsome son flirting with girls, our gregarious son hanging with friends, our carefree son riding his bike down the street. But now these reveries were excruciating reminders of what would never be. I began entertaining shameful fantasies, wishing he would vanish, or imagining he'd get kidnapped or hit by a car. If something like that happened, it wouldn't be our fault, and we'd be free of the curse that had disabled our child and wrecked our lives. Afterward, I'd shudder with guilt, saying, "It's not *his* fault he has mood swings. Hate the disorder, not the child," and so on. But it was hard not to hate everything and everyone: autism, the doctors, the drugs, the school staff, my son, my self—my whole damned life. Les had begun to talk about someday finding a different place for Cam to live, but that possibility seemed years away. What could we do right now?

Cam's second week off meds was a little better, but his moods remained unpredictable and violently polarized.

One of the worst episodes occurred at gymnastics. Since the awful incident the previous fall, he'd done well at his lessons. But this day, early in the no-meds regime, Cam couldn't settle. First he fixated—for the hundredth time—on Coke, but I didn't think he really wanted a Coke. Wrong: as soon as I refused him, he exploded—pinching and slapping me, shouting, pounding the floor. After several minutes, Bridget and I were able to calm him somewhat. But as we guided Cam toward the tramp, he gave a loud growl, wrenched my shirt, raked my neck with his nails, and raced back toward the warm-up room.

He stopped to yank Bridget's collar and grab her hair. I stepped between them, repeating, "Calm down, Cam. Everything's all right. Let's go back on the tramp. Don't you want to jump?" He just wrapped his arm around my neck and pinched me below the Adam's apple. When I pushed his hand away, he snapped at my arm.

My arms and face were scored with scratches, my shirt almost torn off. When he drew blood from my left hand, I finally exploded. With a loud "No!" I pushed him to the mat and pinned his arms.

"Stop it! Stop it! Stop it!" I bellowed, my mouth two inches above my son's nose. "You're gonna stay right here until you calm down!" Cam swivelled his head and pitched his shoulders from side to side, desperately trying to throw off the roaring giant who held him captive.

Bridget silently watched from the other side of the room.

When at last I let him up, he charged again, swinging at my face and gouging the hand that tried to deflect his blows. Only by dancing backward like a boxer did I elude him.

At last Cam collapsed on the floor. Bridget helped me coax the bawling boy to the swing at the center of the room, then we retreated to a corner.

Panting, blotchy, sitting on the floor, I croaked, "Wow. That was bad. I don't know what got into him."

She gently replied, "Well, whatever it was, he'll get over it. But will Dad get over it?" I smiled wanly, unable to speak. I wished I'd let him keep hitting me.

Dr. Cohen wasn't sure how to proceed. He finally floated the possibility of Luvox, an antianxiety medication.

"Well, he's certainly anxious," I said, "so maybe we should give it a try."

At first it did help: Cam was calmer and even napped the day we started it. We breathed a cautious sigh of relief: maybe the crisis was ending. But within days, the imp was back. One report from school gave proof: 124 aggressions; eight biting attempts, two trips to the resource room.

"124 aggressions in a single day," I said to Les. "How is that even possible?"

That evening showed how: Cameron was a dervish. He giggled, ran back and forth down the hall, jumped on his bed and trampoline, spun till he careened into the walls. Then it dawned on us: Luvox is an antidepressant. He was definitely not depressed! Nor was he sleepy; he was so wound up that we had to give him melatonin at bedtime for the first time in three years.

Luvox wasn't the answer.

In the past month, we'd given Cam three medications; one had caused serious side effects and the other two had made him worse. I thought we should take him off meds permanently. At least that way we'd know that the cause of his explosions wasn't some mysterious biochemical agent.

Cohen, too, was ready to throw up his hands; he suggested we bring in another doctor for consultation. We made an appointment at the institute, and in the meantime—another traumatic week—Cam remained med-free.

By the time of our appointment, Les and I had battle scars: she wore a three-inch scratch mark on her right arm bisecting a large, doughnut-shaped bruise. I sported a four-fingers-wide bruise on my left forearm that was actually two bruises, one purple and the other turning green and yellow, both where Cam had bitten me (without breaking the skin) several days apart. These were only the visible marks; the bruises to our psyches were far worse.

Dr. Cohen introduced us to Dr. Matilda Rodriguez, a short, roundish woman with wispy light brown hair. As we described the past few weeks, she met our desperate appeals with mild dark eyes framed by thick, circular glasses. Then, in a soft voice tinged by a faint Hispanic accent, she outlined three possibilities: alpha-agonists such as Clonidine—a blood-pressure medication with a sedating and calming effect; mood stabilizers such as Depakote; major tranquilizers such as Thorazine.

Tranquilizers didn't seem appropriate since they could also cause tardive dyskinesia, which was why we were in this mess in the first place. Depakote, Cohen noted, might be very effective. "With that one, though," Dr. Rodriguez observed, "we'd have to get liver function tests, because it can cause liver damage or pancreatitis. It's rare, but I have to tell you that it's possible. The other drawback is that it can take up to eight weeks to start working."

Liver damage! Pancreatitis! Les and I looked at each other and gulped.

"We have seen lots of kids who were helped by Clonidine. And if it sedates him too much, there's another one, Tenex, that has a milder sedating effect.

Now with these, we can't take him off the medications abruptly, because there's a rebound effect."

"Rebound?"

"If we remove the medication too quickly, his blood pressure could rise very rapidly." She hesitated. "Maybe even dangerously."

This was a lot of information to digest, so Dr. Rodriguez printed out descriptions of the drugs and asked us to call her back in a few days with our decision.

"Bunny, these drugs scare me to death," Les said to me that Friday.

"Me too. 'Would you prefer the high blood pressure or the liver damage?'" I shook my head and stared out the window. Once again the thought of abstaining from all medications crossed my mind—but only briefly. Our scarred arms were ample evidence that *that* method wouldn't work.

Eventually we decided on Clonidine: it would work quickly and its side effects weren't potentially life threatening. We gave Cam his first dose on April 29, almost three years to the day after we'd first given him Risperdal and nearly overdosed him.

There was no immediate change. In fact, the next day, as the school bus pulled up, the driver motioned to me. "Cameron's havin' a rough time, been cryin' for about the last ten minutes."

I walked down the aisle to my wailing son—stripped to his shorts, face patchy, hair disheveled.

"Buddy, what's wrong? You're home now. Let's put your pants back on and go in the house."

Cam continued to cry and rock. His face wore an expression we'd learned to dread—wild eyes and grimacing mouth—the face of a trapped animal. The matron reached down to unfasten his harness, jerking back her hand when Cam swung at her.

"Don't put yourself in harm's way. I'll do it," I cautioned her. As I moved to unstrap him, he clawed at my shirt. I managed to unhook the harness and guide him toward the front. But three rows from the front, Cam darted to the right and snatched the hair of a six-year-old boy.

"Cam! No!!" I shouted. The matron squawked, making spastic, panicky gestures. The driver, a hefty woman in a gray T-shirt, unhooked her seat belt and trotted back to help. The sight of these adults converging on him only increased Cam's panic; he slapped me repeatedly, scratched my face, tried to butt me. The little boy's deafening wails added to the pandemonium.

Once we pried Cam's hand from the boy's hair, I hustled my screaming son into the house, locked him in his room, and inspected the damage. My glasses were twisted, my shirt was torn in two, and my neck was covered with scratches. But these were nothing compared to my emotional state. No doubt Cam felt even worse.

The bus driver brought his school bag to the driveway. "I don't know what got into him!" she said. "He's been having good rides for the last few weeks."

My chest felt like a steamer trunk was sitting on it. I could only choke out, "I'm sorry. We're having a really tough time."

I couldn't bring myself to let Cam out of his room. Instead I sat on the couch with my head in my hands. "God, he could have really hurt that boy!" Then another thought pushed it aside: "Poor Cam. Something is bothering him and he can't tell us what it is."

A couple of hours later the driver called to tell me that they wouldn't allow Cam to ride the bus again until we worked out a new protocol at the IEP meeting, scheduled for Thursday. This incident was Cam's mayday call, and it became ours as well. We'd been talking vaguely for months about someday "seeking a residential placement." Now we realized—or rather I realized, since Les had already faced what I could not—that we'd arrived at the moment of decision. The professionals at the IEP meeting were going to recommend that we move Cam to a new school where he'd live full time. And we were going to agree.

From a Distance

When you consider placing your child in a residence or institution, the guilt that has been a constant nagging presence in your life suddenly starts shouting. You have given up, it says. You are a coward. You have failed your child: the newborn who, not so long ago, you watched take his first breath; the baby whose diapers you changed and whose first words you celebrated; the child you tickled, put to bed, bathed, fed, kissed, nursed, comforted, suffered with, laughed with—the helpless being who relies on you for everything. You are one of *those parents,* the kind you've always sneered at—those too weak to prevail over adversity, the selfish ones who *abandon* their own flesh and blood.

Painful questions assail you. What if somebody hurts him? What if he's neglected, molested, malnourished? Who'll recite "Wynken, Blynken, and Nod" to him? Who'll know which videos and CDs he likes, which foods he prefers? Who will know what he's trying to say?

Nor could I stop hearing Cam's questions—questions more agonizing because he couldn't even ask them. "Who are these people? Where are Mommy and Daddy?"

I could barely admit even to myself the other feeling my thoughts inspired: relief.

The next day I called my sister, who has always been empathetic and intuitive. Perceptive as ever (though not too tactful), she voiced fears I'd not yet even shared with her. "Gee," she said, "will he feel abandoned? Will he think you don't love him?" I pictured Cam whimpering, alone in a strange room. I burst into tears.

As I sobbed, she consoled me with words I hadn't been able to hear from anyone else, including myself: "You can't live like this. His aggression has gotten worse and worse, and he's big. He needs to be someplace where they can do more for him—he needs twenty-four-hour structure. And you guys have done a lot, my God! You found a good school for him, you've been doing this home therapy program for years, you've spent God knows how much money. You've loved him and provided for him, and you've never gotten much back. You're exhausted—you're emotionally used up and physically worn out. You need a break. You guys need a life, too." But her words didn't erase the feeling that I was betraying my son.

Les was both tougher and more compassionate: she knew we had to put aside stubbornness, denial, our prized independence, and do the right thing for Cam. And the right thing was not to hold onto him; it was to let others help us.

Deep down, I knew Cam hadn't been happy for a long time. I also knew that some parents send their kids away out of shame or fear that they'll have to alter their lifestyle. I felt sure those weren't our reasons. During Cam's camp stay the previous summer, we'd glimpsed a truth we were now seeing in full light: parents' greatest challenge is not loving and caring for their child. It's letting their child go. Would we be strong enough to do it?

Given the riot of emotions that had preceded it, the IEP meeting was anticlimactic. Everyone—from the teacher to the OT to the behavior specialists to the county officials—agreed that Cam needed a different placement. Our next step was to meet with the Local Coordinating Council (LCC)—officials from the various county agencies—who would approve the placement and suggest suitable schools.

There was one rough moment: reading Karen Nestor's psychological and behavioral assessment of Cameron. We knew she had to be harsh to justify the out-of-county placement, but her words still felt like punches in the gut. Here was our son reduced to black and white, a case study in developmental failure.

Her assessment begins kindly: "Cameron is frequently affectionate and shows preference for familiar people and enjoys regular leisure activities such as swimming, skating, jumping, music and videos." After that it's all tough stuff:

he exhibits intense and frequent aggression, very frequent and disruptive . . . self-stimulatory behavior (vocalizations, clapping, tearing and eating materials, shredding clothes and disrobing). Due to his level of anxiety, rapid cycling of mood, intensity of aggression, and complex deficits in executive functioning and communication, treatment for Cameron's maladaptive behaviors has been difficult. . . . He appears bored with teaching strategies that have been effective, but unable to adapt to new ones. . . . He has shown periods of improved behavior, but [has] never [been] aggression free. Frequency data accumulated since 1998 indicate rate per-hour quarterly averages ranging from 1.31 to 7.64. . . . Cameron relies on a rigid, predictable schedule and has almost no ability to delay gratification. He over-generalizes the few understandable vocal words he has, making any reliable assessment or treatment of his communication ineffective. He exhibits a highly intensive, labile mood state. For example, he shows manic-like behaviors, such as loud vocalizations, jumping, rapid jerky activity for periods ranging from minutes to hours, then shows aggression, crying and destruction of the environment, indicating anxiety.

The paragraph's last sentence says everything: "it is no longer safe to be alone with him."

The report's final words are startling in their emotionless presentation of our plight: "a 24-hour structured environment with trained available staff is necessary for Cameron's safety, the safety of his family, and for the intense treatment environment needed for potential improvement." Potential, but not likely.

We couldn't say she'd written anything untrue. But she'd left out Cam's humanity—his humor, his high spirits, the intelligence that surfaced often enough for all of us to believe in it. And she ignored the most important fact: he acted this way because he was in pain.

Yet beneath the clinical jargon we could glimpse another boy. A strong-willed, theatrical boy needing constant activity. A boy who expresses himself loudly and intensely, who wants to be the center of attention, whenever he isn't walled into a protective cocoon. A boy much like his parents.

To prepare for the upcoming school visits, I made copies of a video taken of Cam at school. Here was Cam under the camera eye—close-up, but from an emotional distance. If that eye was neutral, mine definitely was not, and as I watched the video, my emotions careened from pride to sadness to frustration before settling on a strange form of admiration.

In the first segment, Cam participates in circle time. When asked, "Who wants a turn?" Cam raises his hand in a half wave. He looks up expectantly, then segues into a sleepy stretch.

They count one, two, three and sing the "hello" song, then the teacher squats in front of my son. "Hi, Cameron."

He looks away, then meets her gaze and almost inaudibly says, "Hi."

"How are you?"

"F-f-f-f-fine."

"Good job. Cameron your turn is. . . ."

"F-f-f-f-fini."

As the others sing with the next child, Cam looks around and says "Loo-ee, loo-ee, loo-ee" out of the side of his mouth. "Eeeh!" he adds, pounding the table and plugging his ears. Translation: "When will this be over?"

This compliant Cam frequently swings his head to clear out the cobwebs. I note the date: May 3, the first week of Clonidine, when he was still sedated.

The second segment shows a one-on-one session with Cam's aide, Terry, who faces him across a gray utility table. They are doing discrete-trial therapy, with a penny as the reward for three consecutive right answers. Two pennies earn a break. She places three note cards in front of him, each with a single word on it.

"Give me 'home.'" She pronounces the word slowly. Looking off to the left, Cam grabs the middle card and hands it to her.

"Yay! Good job!" she squeals with mock excitement. "Give me five." Cam rocks, grimaces, slaps five. He vocalizes in a high register, "Uh new, huh!"

Terry points to her nose to prompt him to look at her and sets the cards in front of him again, but he's staring to the right. She nudges his chin, but he still won't look, so she tries an attention-getting tactic: "Do this," she says, clapping twice. He claps once, still gazing off.

"Give me 'home.'" Cam pounds the table, says "Eee wee," then hands her a card. She neutrally rearranges the cards. Cam bites his hand lightly, knowing that no response means he gave a wrong answer. He still hasn't looked at a card.

"Nokay, noooookaaaaayyy," he says into his right hand, then slaps his left elbow. Out of the side of his mouth he says, "Nose?" Or is it "knows?"

Four more requests to touch "home" follow, with only one successful response. Not once does he look at a card. Instead he vocalizes, shifts in his seat, waves his fingers.

"Why doesn't she make him look?" I wonder. But I know the answer: he has no idea what's on the cards, so guessing is as good a strategy as any. Anyone watching the tape will see a child who can barely suppress his tics and stims long enough to glance at a face, a child who knows that if he just tolerates the drill long enough, he'll eventually get to do something else. This child doesn't want to look at "home"; he wants to go home.

Will they also see what I see, that this drill bores him silly? Surely another school will have a better plan.

The third and longest segment, recorded two weeks later, is even more excruciating to watch. Wearing a bright orange knit shirt with a white stripe, Cam sits at his cubicle rocking backward, slapping his own ear, pounding the table, saying, "Huh, ho, hoy."

A voice from behind the camera says sternly, "Cameron, you need to do your work."

He looks around. "Za mooh, za mooh. Ha bu doo, ho bu doo. Za mooths." Cut.

He's outdoors with classmates, raising a parachute over their heads and taking turns going under it. Cam helps raise the chute once, then spends several minutes clapping, thumping himself on the chest, and vocalizing "Too wee, too wee!"

Terry nudges Cam forward. Fingers jammed into his ears, he walks under the parachute, emerges on the other side, then sprints to the far end of the field, claps, sticks his fingers into his ears again, then hunches his shoulders, bracing himself for an adult's inevitable arrival. Faith, Cam's young teacher, retrieves him. He snatches her necklace (why would she wear such a thing to class?), then grabs a small twig and starts smoothing it.

"Haaattt," he says, as Terry and Faith each grab an arm and walk him to a bench.

Next comes T-ball. When Terry pulls him up for his turn, he gouges her hand and assumes his Bartleby mode: he'd prefer not to hit, run, or participate in any way. He'd prefer to kneel on the grass and pluck stems. Terry and Faith count to three, lift him by the armpits, and walk him to the tee: *they* walk, that is—he refuses to let his feet touch the ground.

The PE teacher hands him the bat. Realizing there's no way out, he takes two strong swings that barely graze the ball, which plunks to the ground a foot away. After the third swing—a feeble tap—Terry shouts, "Now run." Cam strolls a few feet, then slaps her hand. When they reach the cone serving as first base, he pauses, chuckles, shakes free, and dashes toward the far end of the field.

Terry fetches him, fighting off his gouges and scratches as he falls to his knees. "Cameron, stand up!" He slaps her and crams his fingers back into his ears. When she tries to pull him up, he raises his feet off the ground in resistance.

"God!" Cam declares.

For several minutes, the aides fruitlessly try to make Cam stop plucking grass and taking off his shoes. Finally it's time to go inside. Cam races to the first small tree and tears off two leaves. When he's pulled away he squeals, stops cold, collapses, lies supine. The aides lift him up and walk him into the school building.

In the epilogue, Cam sits shirtless at his cubicle, Terry behind the half wall to his left. The missing shirt means he has ripped it in anger, and he's still not happy: he has to complete a foam puzzle consisting of the numerals from 1 to 9. He turns in his chair and shouts, "Pumm yea, pudya," gesturing and biting the back of the chair.

He takes a piece: "Ah pun yeah, pudja," he exclaims with a grimace. He inserts a piece, looks down at his right hand, says "Hair," then "Whackya zak," as he places another piece in.

"Dwayyah!" he shouts.

"Cam, do your work," Terry says.

"This old man!" he half growls, half sings. "Eeeh!" He slaps the table.

She shows him his *Blue's Clues* boombox. "Do you wanna work . . ."

"Top ahhh!" he interrupts, slapping his left arm.

"Do puzzle for Blue," she says, handing him the "6" piece and pointing to the puzzle.

"No, no hoops," he says. He twists the piece: is it a 6 or 9? Pounding the table, he hollers, "Dan ya hone, own ya way, sheh! Oon da, oon dah!"

"Finish puzzle," she says, "for Blue."

"Reen ya go!" he says, picking up another piece and putting it in. "You ta kay, you ta kay!" He puts two more pieces in. "Un ya pwash! Eh, ya!"

The video mercifully ends.

It's a pretty fair exhibit of Cam's behaviors. I felt proud that he paid attention during circle time and marveled at his ability to manipulate his teacher.

Painful though it was to watch the two cubicle segments (all those twitches and tics!), they were also a revelation, for I was able to decipher phrases that, in person, sounded like gibberish. I recognized "za mooth" from *The Little Mermaid,* when the singing crab says, "The mood." Was Cam saying he wasn't in the mood to work? "Dan ya hone, on ya weh" might have been something like "on the way home." It's afternoon, so perhaps he was wondering if it was time to go home. "Reenyago," *in you go;* "pudya," *puzzle;* "no hoops," *no help;* "Tap aah!" *stop it* (spoken to the aide tormenting him). And "This Old Man" is, of course, a counting song: was he associating the numerical puzzle with the song? The teachers didn't respond to anything he said. No wonder he was mad.

This, I thought, was why we had to find a different school.

In the outdoor segment, I saw again the boy who lived half in looking-glass land. The fingers in the ears blocked out demands but may also have blocked sounds others couldn't hear. Perhaps a car engine three blocks away drowned out the birds he wanted to hear, or maybe the birds themselves bothered him. Most of all I was saddened by the graphic dramatization of Cam's difference, of the estrangement that endures even when he's with others. Leavening my frustration, however, was admiration for my son's spirit. He resisted playing ball for almost twenty minutes, never once yielding unless physically forced or offered a reward. You might dub this "autistic resistance." But it was also a principled refusal. And it earned him attention and power. The others had to respond!

I saw two other people quite clearly in the video. In my son's defiance, I detected my own stubbornness. And through the fun-house mirror of his autism, I witnessed an ordinary kid refusing to be pushed around. Would strangers see this Cam? Or would they see only "noncompliance," "highly intensive mood state with rapid cycles," "complex deficits in executive functioning and communication," and "very frequent and disruptive levels of self-stimulatory behavior?"

Biting Time

The LCC meeting was set for June 6. The days passed in a blur of worry, then froze as we anticipated four more months of Cam's aggression and mood swings. We were biding time, but time was not biding us; it was chewing us up and spitting us out. Again.

To complicate matters, Cam's sleep problems were back, even though Clonidine was supposed to sedate him. One night we woke at 2:30 to hear Cam singing "Old McDonald," after which he bounded out of bed, having peed all over Bernie and his blanket. He jumped, clapped, hollered, sang, and growled; he leaped on the trampoline and couch; he pounded on the walls. Our little house had been spun in a time machine; it was 1996 again.

The next evening he couldn't get to sleep. At 10:30, I put him to bed for the third time. "Bwinken nod," he requested.

Tired and irritable, I refused. He locked his hands onto my left arm, then grabbed my shirt.

"Cam, go to sleep," I pleaded, gently and then angrily. As my voice rose, Les came running. The encounter escalated as she tried to pull me away. Cam wouldn't release his grip; I wouldn't back off. She tried to wrestle me off Cam's bed. I wouldn't move. We reached a stalemate, although that word, which suggests stasis, doesn't do justice to the three flushed, panting people in the room.

The same scenario replayed itself twice more in the next few days. It seemed we were all trapped in a time warp or in some autistic ritual.

On May 22 after Cam got off the bus, I joined him at the maple tree he was plucking.

"How ya doin,' buddy?" I asked. "Did you have a good day?"

A brief whine, then his hand snaked out and ripped a large hole in my T-shirt.

"Come on. Take it easy, now." As I tried to detach his hands from my shirt, he bit me hard on the inside of my right forearm.

"Ow! Shit!"

Cam looked surprised that he'd bitten into living flesh and not a glove or toy.

For a moment I stared in horror at the bluish, bloody half-circle throbbing on my forearm. Then I yanked his hands from my shirt, hustled him into the house, shoved him into his bedroom, slammed and locked his door.

Stunned, I regarded my arm, which looked like one of those gummy inserts dentists use to measure for a new crown. Blood seeped from the bluish crescent. This was by far my worst bite yet. And this time I'd definitely done nothing to bring it on.

I fetched a bag of frozen peas from the freezer and placed it on the mark, then called my doctor's office. A nurse told me I'd have to go to the emergency room to get the bite cleaned and treated. She admonished me, "Human mouths are even dirtier than dogs.' If it got infected, it could get bad. You might even lose your arm." Why she was lecturing me? Did she think I'd *tried* to get bitten?

I could hardly go to the ER with Cam, and it wasn't possible to leave him at home. I paced, then rang Leslie's cell phone. No answer. Dana, our therapist, wasn't due for another hour. What to do? Did I need a tetanus shot? A hepatitis shot? A tourniquet?

I finally called the ER at St. Giles. In three minutes I spoke to three different people, the last of whom referred me to an "urgent care" facility. I called one.

"Hello. I've got a bite on my arm that broke the skin. Do I need a shot of some kind?"

"Sir, I can't give medical advice over the phone. You're welcome to come in and take your turn to see our doctor."

"You can't even tell me what the usual procedures are for treating a bloody bite?" I was getting irritated. How complicated could this be?

"No, sir, I'm afraid you'll have to come in and see what the doctor says."

I hung up and called my doctor back. The office was closed. I left a message and in five minutes the nurse returned my call.

"Did you just call Dr. Wagner?"

"Yes."

"And didn't you just talk to us about ten minutes ago?"

"Yes, that was me."

"And didn't I tell you to go to the emergency room?"

"Yes, you did."

"Then why are you calling us back again?"

"The staff at the ER told me I didn't need to go there. And you know as well as I do that I'd just sit around for hours anyway."

I actually chuckled. But why was I was being cross-examined like a ten-year-old caught shoplifting? Suddenly I understood: other than bums or drunks, who ever gets bitten by another human? I explained that it wasn't some barfly who'd bitten me but my eleven-year-old son. Her tone softening at once, the nurse advised me to drop in the next morning for a tetanus shot.

I found Cam lying on his bed, his mouth turned down, his pants wet. Did the pants explain the bite? Or was it a delayed reaction to recent events? It was easy to forget that Cam was feeling even worse than we were: he was the one whose senses and emotions were being tossed like leaves in a tempest. If time seemed jagged and jumpy to us, it could only have been worse for him.

The next day, a disturbing realization lingered: for the first time, Cameron had actually hurt me. Clearly the new placement couldn't wait.

Counsel

As we drove to our meeting with the Local Coordinating Council, I pleaded with Les not to cry: "You'll make me blubber right along with you."

She promised to be stoic.

As we entered the room, I glanced at the six strangers sitting around the oval table, none of whose names stayed with me for three seconds. Were they friends or foes? What did they want from us?

For many years we'd dealt by phone or e-mail with Mary Kate Rota, the head of county special ed, but we'd never met her in person. She turned out to be a diminutive woman with small features and baby-blue eyes, her long graying hair forming an odd contrast to her doll-like face. She reminded the others that we'd struggled mightily to provide an "appropriate educational environment" for Cameron, but that his aggression and behaviors had finally made it impossible. Our case sounded desperate, even to me.

When she asked about our home life, I looked at Les, whose eyes were welling up: she'd already broken her promise. I intended to describe Cam's aggression and mood swings, maybe even show them the bite mark, and say, "We don't want to do this. It's hard to admit that you can't handle your own child, but we've finally realized that he'll do better somewhere else." But as I reached "admit," I suddenly foresaw Cameron's empty bedroom. I couldn't continue.

Two of the women were also getting wet eyes. It seemed they weren't enemies.

Rota was skillful. The county and state didn't want to pay for our son to attend an expensive out-of-state school. But after reviewing the various facilities in Maryland, she said offhandedly, "Why don't we go ahead and look at out-of-state facilities as well?" In other words, she expected every Maryland school to reject Cam, and she was smoothing the way for the inevitable out-of-state placement.

Nobody offered a single objection. For the rest of the meeting, in fact, they spoke to us gently, as if we were made out of rare china and might shatter at the first loud noise. But no one made eye contact. They felt sorry for us but didn't want to get too close. At the end of the meeting, Rota patted Les on the back and told us we were doing the right thing.

Why, then, were we still so frightened and sad?

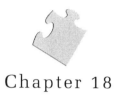

Chapter 18

Departures

All places that the eye of heaven visits
Are to a wise man ports and happy havens.
Teach thy necessity to reason thus:
There is no virtue like necessity.
—Shakespeare, *Richard II*

"It'll be like sending your kid off to college," a helpful friend said to me after he heard we were looking for a residential school for Cam. His son had just finished his freshman year.

"Yeah, I guess so," I replied, smiling tightly. Except that his son was a self-possessed young man of eighteen, and mine was twelve and functioned at the level of a three-year-old.

The coming summer would be an odyssey of visits to prospective schools, each one foreshadowing Cam's own departure. We avoided dwelling on the future by filling the days organizing packets of psychological and educational assessments, copying documents and videos, phoning schools, and making travel arrangements. We vowed to ask probing questions, present Cam fairly, and evaluate each place dispassionately. But the decision was not up to us alone: a school also had to choose Cam. And given his behaviors, linguistic and social deficits, and cognitive impairment, he would be a tough sell.

The process was also fraught with ambivalence: I hoped to find the right school for Cam, yet a part of me hoped we wouldn't. I didn't want to lose my son.

Hugging the Shore

The Callaway Carver staff had made it abundantly clear that Cam was one of the most difficult children they'd ever met. We doubted that any Maryland school would accept him, and looked on the first visits as dry runs for the real tests: the more intensive facilities out of state.

In mid-May, we drove 85 miles to a farming district on Maryland's Eastern Shore to visit Three Sisters School. The Baltimore County officials had called it "Maryland's premiere school for special needs students." So why didn't their website and literature even mention autism?

The long driveway leading to the fifty-acre campus brought us past a convent, chapel, and suite of offices. Pungent odors of loam and cow manure assailed us as we stepped from the car. At the door we were welcomed by Carla Thomas, a friendly, freckled lady who gave a quick rundown of their programs and accompanied us as we dropped in on a classroom.

A teenager named Eddie silently shook our hands again and again, then clapped and drew us into the room. As Eddie prompted me to clap with him, Les helped a cute twelve-year-old girl fold socks. Two other students held Dyna Mites—small electronic communication devices displaying a menu of icons and pictures. The students touched the picture and the device pronounced the word. Wouldn't one of these be perfect for Cam?

Each student shared one of the attractive dorm rooms—a little smaller than Cam's bedroom at home—with another student. I wondered how Cam's roommate would like his constant bouncing, shredding, bedwetting, and sporadic insomnia.

Three Sisters had everything: a large, heated swimming pool; a big gym and spacious, modern playground; even a greenhouse, garden, and café where older students learned trades. We visited a large room where a group of adults performed light assembly tasks. Nobody was running around, nobody was disruptive. How would Cam fit into this subdued environment? Carla assured us that they'd seen every type of behavior problem in their thirty-plus-year history, but we saw no sign of any behaviors remotely like Cam's. I feared he'd cut a swath through this place in a matter of hours.

But the longer we stayed, the more we liked it. We were impressed by the clean, comprehensive layout and the caring atmosphere. And here the hands-on staff weren't twenty-somethings fresh out of college, but seasoned veterans. This school seemed at once tranquil and industrious—nearly enchanted, as if a higher power had dropped this haven for the exceptional in the middle of nowhere.

We were positive they'd never accept Cam.

Before making any further school visits, I had to travel to Boston for a professional conference. The day before I was to leave, I packed while Cam worked with his therapist. Folding my sport coat into the suitcase, I recalled an incident from the previous fall when I'd driven to College Park for a one-day conference. Les had been visiting her family in Montana, so I'd left Cam with Rachel, a teacher at his school we'd just hired.

At the lunch break, I'd called to check on them. Rachel breathed heavily into the phone. She was overwrought. "He attacked me. He charged like a bull!" she said shrilly. "He pinched and gouged my hand and tried to choke me. He grabbed my hair and wouldn't let go. I couldn't get him off." Her voice quaked.

I cringed as I pictured Rachel, who stood about five feet tall and weighed maybe 110 pounds, trying to fend off my strapping son.

"Did you try to give him something to eat?"

"Yes. At first I thought he was hungry, but then he went after me again. I held him off." She paused to catch her breath. "He kept saying 'hone, hone.'"

"Hone": with his mom gone for the weekend, Cam needed me there. In the past I'd left him for a few hours with sitters when Les was out of town, but this time he couldn't handle my absence. I'd made a huge mistake.

But I hadn't given my paper yet, so I told Rachel to take Cam to the playground and assured her I'd be "hone" as soon as I possibly could. After a hasty rundown of my talk, I raced back to Baltimore with a colleague, breaking every speed limit on the way.

We opened our back door to find Rachel in the kitchen, wiping away tears with a tissue. Her face was blotchy; her arms were scored with scratches. She managed to choke out her story: Cam had attacked her again at the playground, so she'd retreated to the car until he'd calmed down enough to go home. Then she'd locked him in his room.

I apologized and sent her home. My colleague, bless him, didn't show the horror he must have felt.

Rachel had originally agreed to work on Sunday also, but when she returned the next day, she told me she couldn't work with Cam. "I'm afraid he's going to hurt me. When I couldn't get him off me, I realized that he was bigger and stronger than me." Her lower lip quivered.

I felt awful. It was my fault for entrusting Cam to an inexperienced sitter, my fault for not preparing both of them better. I felt as though I was the one who had beaten her up.

As I gazed down at my packed suitcase this May, I realized I couldn't make my trip. If Cam injured Les while I was away, I'd never forgive myself. There would be other conferences.

The Wallbrook School, in a DC suburb, provided a stark contrast to Three Sisters. The campus consisted of a cramped, fenced playground and a single building locked up like a prison. We had to stand outside a heavy double door and ring a bell for admittance; every wing was walled off from the others. Our initial misgivings only multiplied during the visit.

A heavyset woman named Nancy gave us the tour. In one classroom, a boy about Cam's age, his eyes glassy from medication, worked on a number-recognition drill. Lids drooping, he scanned the numbers and tapped out the sum; between tasks he laid his head down on the table. So this was how they handled noncompliant students: drug them into oblivion.

The room had one set of bins and one table. There was no schedule, no art-work, no calendar; there were certainly no electronic communication devices, and when we asked Nancy about them, she answered vaguely, "Oh, many of our kids carry a book to communicate."

In a second class, a half-dozen students of various ages ran aimlessly around. One staff person (whom we soon realized was deaf) signed to us (according to Nancy) that an irate student was trying to run away. Three staff members blocked the door while the other students shouted excitedly, hopped up and down, covered their ears, and screamed.

We didn't linger. After we escaped, I stole a glance at Les, who was obviously thinking the same thing I was: "How could anyone get an education here?" It's not unusual for an autistic child to "elope," as they call it. But why was one student allowed to disrupt the entire class? Was anyone in charge here?

Nancy didn't take us to the homes—that would have required a separate visit. But we learned that the students lived in ordinary neighborhoods, four to a home, which were staffed one-to-one from 2:30 to 10:30.

"What do the kids do after school?" Leslie asked.

"Some do IEP work." This seemed to mean that they continued their school day: not comforting, given what we'd seen in the classes. "Every home has a big yard, and each student has their own room. Some of the kids have a TV/VCR combo, and they watch TV at night." She thought this was just dandy.

On the drive home, we discussed the visit.

"'They watch TV at night.' Good Lord, if we just wanted Cam to watch TV all night, we wouldn't need a residential school!" Les said.

"Educational objective: Cameron will learn to be a couch potato. And how about that mob scene in the classroom? Who in the world would send their kid there?"

"People who don't know any better or don't care."

"Or don't have any choice." But we had a choice, and we weren't sending our son here.

We hoped to find a suitable place nearby but knew it would be foolish to eliminate good schools, no matter how far away. And one distant prospect came on strong: the Bright Spirit School, located in Kansas. As it happened, their admissions director, Joseph Woodward, was coming to Baltimore to interview other potential clients, so we arranged a home visit. A tall, sharply dressed African American in his thirties, Woodward offered a well-oiled sales pitch and responded thoughtfully to my queries. His presence was a siren call: for a few moments, I felt like the dad of a star high school athlete being wooed by recruiters.

He videotaped Cam as I outlined his aggression, stims, rigidity. But when he asked, "What's with the pacifier? Is that a regular thing with him?" I heard criticism, and for the rest of the visit couldn't let down my guard. But it really didn't matter, for one fact overshadowed Woodward's glowing description of the school.

"I'll be honest," I told him. "We're concerned that Bright Spirit is so far away."

He told me about a family who'd chartered a jet to fly their daughter there and another who'd rented an RV. They advised parents to prepare kids by going to the airport and coming back, then making another trip only to board the plane, then another to finally get airborne.

"You'd be surprised," he said. "Some kids you'd never think could fly end up liking it."

I pictured Cam in coach class, rocking violently and kicking the seat in front of him, kneeling in the aisle while shredding a string, belching loudly, and shouting, "Day-O"!

I imagined the dagger glares of the other passengers. I heard the pilot radio Des Moines, asking to be cleared for an emergency landing. I saw attendants clutching the backs of our shirts, hustling us down the aisles and thrusting the three of us out the hatch onto the tarmac.

"No flying!" screams Raymond Babbitt. For good reason.

I scheduled a visit to Bright Spirit anyway. They couldn't see us until August, and I hoped (I can't say I believed) that we'd have found a school by then. But we had to keep our options open: Bright Spirit might be our only choice.

The next week, my mother, Lois, came for a long-scheduled visit and volunteered to accompany me to the next school, Shelter Beach.

Unlike Wallbrook, where nobody seemed to be in charge, this place (or places—we had to drive to three different sites) was professionally run and well organized. Both the residential director, Linda Brass, a tanned redhead, and the educational director—a heavy, gray-haired lady with a warm smile—impressed us as competent and smart.

As she drove us around in her Jeep Cherokee, Brass told us she'd observed Cam at Callaway Carver the previous week, when he'd been on his best behavior.

"He was great. He followed directions and went right along with everybody. He seemed very happy."

Ha, I thought: if he were happy, I wouldn't be here.

She drove us to a neat beige ranch house where Cam would bunk with one other boy in a residence for five. It seemed clean, but the backyard contained no play equipment and plenty of shrubs: easy pickings for Cam. How would they avoid the same problems we faced at home?

We were scheduled to visit the school, so I was surprised when we pulled up to a strip mall. Then I realized with dismay that this *was* the school, wedged into a few rooms between Miller's Liquor Store and the Chesapeake Diner. A two-lane highway ran about twenty-five yards from the front door. As I got out of the Jeep, I had disturbing visions of Cam dashing in front of a speeding truck.

The four classrooms were tiny and shabby. In one, an enormous teenager matched number-words to numerals, and a helmeted boy worked a twelve-piece puzzle. In another we met two of Cam's potential roommates. One rocked in lotus position on the floor; the other dully fingered yarn. I wondered which educational goals they were fulfilling.

In the third room, a chubby, blonde girl with bright red cheeks spotted us, giggled, and hopped toward us, gleefully proffering her mechanical communication device. She asked for and received hugs. Then we met Jimmy, a fourteen-year-old with chopped-off sandy hair, who glanced up from his arithmetic and declared in a surprising bass, "Lois and Mark? I thought you said 'Lois and Clark,'" then slapped his knee and chortled. We chatted with Jimmy for several minutes. What was this guy doing here?

The room at the end of the corridor housed the kind of children who don't appear in promotional brochures: a blonde girl with severe cerebral palsy, a non-ambulatory middle-schooler being fed through a tube, a child of indeterminate age strapped onto a device to help straighten the spine. The residential director kept up a steady patter while we stood uncomfortably in the room. We didn't stay long.

The school had no playground or gym, no occupational therapy room, no speech clinic, no music room—not even a dining hall. We couldn't find fault with the pleasant, conscientious staff. They were trying hard and seemed to care about the kids. But the physical setup was a disgrace. The State of Maryland deemed this an adequate facility for their neediest children? Brass and the ed director hastened to assure us that they'd just signed a contract to have a new school built; they even showed us the floor plan. In two or three years, I thought, this place might be decent. But that was too late for us.

Les and I had gradually adjusted to the idea that Cameron was disabled. Even so, this place had shocked me: the children with misshapen heads, obese girls with rampant acne, preteens with tremors, boys in threadbare, ill-fitting clothes who drooled or gazed toward us blankly. On the hour's drive home, I couldn't join in my mom's bright chatter: I felt as if a curtain had been lifted upon the world of the institutionalized—an underworld where parents deposit children they want to forget.

For the next few days, I was haunted by the sense that I'd accidentally glimpsed something dirty. "Normal" people seemed phony, their lives built on a willful blindness to the suffering of those with twisted bodies or blunted brains. How could I take part in such a lie? How could I cast my only son into this land of the forgotten?

The prospects for placing Cam nearby looked dim. Three Sisters was geared for higher-functioning students; Wallbrook was chaotic; Shelter Beach was a shame. Yet all three schools were interested in him, and Shelter Beach was downright enthusiastic. If they accepted him, we might have to go to court to prove it wasn't suitable. It was time to stop hugging the shore and launch our boat toward distant ports.

Wonderland Revisited

Cam had done so well at Camp Wonder—and Les and I had so relished the break—that we didn't hesitate to take him back in 2001.

We were met at the camp by a young man named Billy, who stood about 4' 8" and weighed at least 180 lbs. He could have been anywhere between fifteen and twenty-five years old. In a high-pitched voice, he repeatedly asked single-word questions—"Carry?" "Car?"—while helping me unload Cam's gear. He too wanted to shake hands again and again, saying "hi" and "good-bye" each time. Billy understood the concept of obligation: since he'd helped me, he felt I owed him some pushes on the large, bench-like swing Cam had so loved the previous summer.

Billy seemed high-functioning. But when Les tried to converse with him, the dialogue was right out of *Alice in Wonderland*.

"Where is home?" she asked.

"Where my mommy is."

"And where is your mommy?"

"At home."

She tried again; same results. It was hard to fault his logic: what else does "home" mean?   Cam knew where *he* was, and swaggered around like a big man on campus, strolling along the trail to the cabins and stripping branches from trees as if he owned the place. In the mess hall where we waited to register, he sat patiently and came immediately when we called.

The boy ahead of us in line looked non-disabled, said "Hi," and talked to his father about his plans for the week. But this first impression was also deceptive, as we learned when his parents unpacked a pharmacy full of medications from a metal briefcase. Sorting through the drugs, they exuded a weary pride, as if the many medications verified their diligence and love.

Our instructions to the nurse were simple: make sure Cam swallowed his Clonidine pills.

Nearby was Teddy who, like Cam, had grown a few inches and slimmed down. Cam hopped excitedly as they played a clapping game. But Teddy was scheduled to be a "floater" this year, which meant that Cam's aide would be Missy, a square, fresh-faced girl with curly, light brown hair.

My first words to her were "Better watch the hair." Perhaps I was a touch abrupt: I didn't approve of their decision to change Cam's aide. No doubt we frightened the poor girl to death with our litany of instructions and warnings.

As I glanced from my bright-eyed son in his cool denim shorts and mesh muscle shirt to the other campers—gnomish Billy, a man with CP who kept imitating Cam's claps—I felt a mixture of pride, anxiety, and hope. In his own way, my son was catching up with old pals, checking out the rookies, establishing himself as a vet. For an instant I was staggered by a flash of Cameron without autism, and caught myself asking again: is he one of us or one of them? Is there really a difference?

No portentous thunderstorm commemorated this year's departure, only a buzzing blend of apprehension, numbness, and relief. But there was one other change from the previous year, and it was monumental: Camp Wonder was no longer just a break; it was a trial run for the longer separation to come. In the car, Les began to cry softly. I too felt a gigantic void open in my heart.

Ministries of Love

We visited two schools that weekend. First stop: the Laurels, part of the Blair Psychological Institute. Located in an affluent suburb amidst self-consciously "quaint" shops and the obligatory Starbucks, it was an impressive-looking place, all red brick and ivy. But again appearances were deceiving.

The Laurels consisted of three separate small buildings, entered through an electronically locked room opening onto an enclosed courtyard. Inside, inmates lived under the camera's Cyclopean eye twenty-four hours a day, seven days a week. Blank-eyed technicians incessantly compiled data. With a frown I recalled our experiences with Callaway's endless data collecting.

Our gregarious guide informed us that the Laurels was not a school but a clinic for kids with severe behavior problems. As she chattered, we watched a boy with the bruises of a chronic head banger being repeatedly helped from the floor, then flopping back down again. In another room, a small girl ("she bites, scratches, hits—you name it") flung soggy Cheerios.

Our guide explained that kids stayed here only six months and then went to a "discharge site" or home. Again I frowned, this time at the prospect of having to repeat our search next year. There was no reason to stay: we needed a permanent solution, and this wasn't it.

We understood the need for locks and intensive behavior management; even so, this place gave us the creeps. The constant surveillance, the sense that it was a laboratory rather than a residence, and the disturbing condition of the kids made us feel we'd stumbled into some sinister Orwellian social experiment. It was both too intense and too clinical.

Les commented, "It's Callaway all over again."

"Only worse."

"And it was filthy," she concluded.

At the Danner School in rural Pennsylvania, a personable young social worker named Brenda showed us the attached "villa" where Cam would live. We chuckled as one young man carefully scrutinized us, then marched to the TV and flipped through the channels with a practiced air. Finally he tuned the set to a cartoon channel and sank down on the couch to watch. The channel was so staticky that you could barely make out the figures, yet he and two other teenagers stared at it intently as though the picture were sharp. Was this was how they perceived things, as if through a dense fog? The ghostly images seemed to illustrate the boys' position in the world, where they were treated as incomplete outlines of "real" people.

The blurry TV picture also defined the shabby condition of this school, where the back door opened onto a weed-grown asphalt playground ("we're going to fix that," Brenda assured us) that resembled a drug-infested, inner-city park. A sense of weariness pervaded the place; the very walls seem to groan, "Don't expect much."

Both places depressed us deeply: a prison and a warehouse. The word "institution," with its ugly connotations of incarceration and impersonality, seemed all too apt. We knew our son was "severely" autistic (one step up from "profound," in official classifications), but he didn't belong in either place.

Five days into Cam's stay, Leslie fielded a call from the camp nurse, who tactfully informed her, "Cam is presenting quite a few problems." He wouldn't sleep and wouldn't eat. He was attacking staff and couldn't sit still. "It's as if he's charged by electricity," she said. His yelling, clapping, and chest beating were driving everyone crazy.

Not even a week had passed, and the end of camp seemed imminent. Yet the nurse recommended that we stick it out. "He's safe here," she said, "and you guys can get a break. Don't let your guilt take advantage of you! Go take a long bath!"

She asked us if they could give Cam Benadryl to help him sleep. Dr. Rodriguez recommended instead that we add a half dose of Clonidine in the afternoon—the extra dose we'd been resisting administering for a month. We agreed to it.

That day the Danner School called to reject Cam: he was too severe for them. We didn't care—we'd already rejected them—but the news didn't make us any happier.

The next day, a Friday, I drove 290 miles to visit another school in Virginia. Ten minutes after I left, the place was a blur in my mind. The school personnel were all starting to look alike: women with bright smiles masking desperation. This place thankfully lacked the jail-like atmosphere of the Laurels or Wallbrook, but its small building was nearly as inadequate as Shelter Beach's.

Three Sisters was looking better and better.

Peering through the rain-drenched windshield as I crept through a cloudburst, I wondered again what would happen if *no* school ended up being right for Cam.

Saturday the camp nurse phoned to tell Les that Cam had torn a staff member's shirt. It seemed doubtful whether our "very, very difficult child" (Dr. R's phrase) would make it through the week. Could we subject them to the continued assault? Could we subject *Cam* to it? We trudged gloomily through the day. Guilt nagged like a toothache. Finally we decided to give it a couple more days to see if the extra medication made any difference. If not, we'd pick him up Tuesday.

Had he been traumatized last year, but the two of us too worn out to notice? And if he couldn't handle camp, how in the world would he ever adjust to a new home?

On Sunday I made more copies of the videotape and created three more packets for the Massachusetts schools I was slated to visit the following week. Suddenly I missed Cam so much that my chest actually ached.

I examined physical proof of his existence: the scar from the bite he'd given me three weeks earlier. Like my memory of the incident, the mark was fading. No longer red and itching, it was becoming a keloid bump, as if my body was overcompensating for the injury by furiously producing new tissue. Fingering the scar, I realized that our preparations for Cam's departure—the copying, the visits, the frequent discussions of his behaviors, "strengths" and "needs"—had actually made us more consumed with him, more anxious about him. Our efforts to heal were producing their own disfigurement.

Scylla and Charybdis

On Wednesday I flew to Providence, then drove to Massachusetts for more school visits. The Massachusetts Institute for Children cultivated an image of success, from its modern, cheerful buildings to the young, attractive admissions officer who led me around. She even gave me directions to other schools, as if to say, "We're so good, we'll even encourage you to assess our competitors."

A walk-through revealed a state-of-the-art, all-ABA school where each student got a daily health check. A team of professionals regularly reviewed each student's progress. Teachers staffed the group homes, which boasted a 1:2 ratio of residents to staff; students could stay there 365 days per year (no built-in vacations, as with Three Sisters and Bright Spirit). They even offered on-site day care for employees! This school was what Callaway Carver dreamed of becoming.

I attended a graduation ceremony for a young man with Down syndrome. Beaming, the graduate thanked everyone and announced, "It took me a while, but I did it."

I was moved: even our wildest dreams didn't include such an event for Cameron.

Yet the ceremony also exposed the MIC's main drawback: their concentration on higher-functioning students. I saw lots of five-, six-, or seven-year-olds who could speak, read, and write, but none like Cam. Near the end of the tour we did briefly visit a "staff-intensive" classroom for lower-functioning students (located, not surprisingly, in the basement). The admissions officer proudly told me that one of the autistic students had enrolled wearing a helmet and long splints on both arms because of his chronic self-injurious behaviors; those were now gone. She also noted that they had a long waiting list for this class: translation, "Don't get your hopes up."

I saw almost no chance of Cam's getting in, even if we could wait eighteen months for an opening, which we couldn't. Walking back to my rental car, I felt a pang of envy for how the other half of the autism spectrum lived. My envy soon soured: sure, the place was outstanding, but if you don't take the tough cases, how much is your success really worth? What happens to more difficult kids?

Answer: other schools pick up the slack, and my next stop was one of them, the Garden Grove Center, a spiffy campus with manicured grounds and a fully equipped playground. Although the admissions officer assured me that they served kids at all levels of ability, every student I saw had a physical disability: one boy couldn't stop drooling and another sat immobile in a complicated, high-tech wheelchair. Though less cuddly and cute, these kids needed more care than the confident six-year-olds merrily blossoming at the MIC. These students, I thought, would blemish the MIC's sparkling image.

The admissions person told me that Cam would be more suited for their Center for Basic Skills than for their Center for Behavioral Development, which, she said, treated children with behaviors even more severe than his. Good Lord: more severe? She didn't go into detail, but from time to time I heard loud thumps and agonized howls from behind the gleaming white walls—the sounds of behavioral development.

With a jolt, I realized that Cam would be among the more capable students here, where kids started prevocational training at ages eleven and twelve and worked at several local businesses. In short, it wasn't a really a school; it was a Center for Basic Skills. The idea seemed to be that if your kid ended up here, you'd already given up on academics, so there was no need to waste time pretending. Sensible, but sobering.

No matter: Garden Grove didn't have an opening. At best, Cam would be wait-listed. But we couldn't wait. Heaving a sigh, I started up the car. Would this trip too be for nothing?

I had a lot to think about on the plane. Clearly, the MIC was little more than a bewitching fantasy. Garden Grove was a more realistic option, but something about the place—maybe it was those howls—left an unpleasant aftertaste. If Cam were less challenging, would an opening have magically appeared?

Slouching gloomily in the cramped plane seat, I felt squeezed between cloudy wishes and hard reality. Well, I thought, maybe the trip wasn't completely worthless: at least I was learning a lot about the range of schools available. I told myself we were fortunate to live on the East Coast, with several schools only a short plane trip away. Pity the poor families in Montana!

When I arrived home, I was surprised to find the front door locked. Then I spotted Cam's duffel bag.

Camp Wonder had called on Thursday and pleaded with Les to fetch Cam. He'd been hitting and biting other campers; everyone was terrified of him. They'd been so eager to get rid of him that they'd driven halfway to Philadelphia to drop him off in a Roy Rogers parking lot.

The ex-camper was thin, tan, and tired. A check of his belongings revealed that he'd departed without his CD player, discs, and beloved Pokemon blanket; with only two of ten pairs of shorts and three of ten shirts; sans sleeping bag (he'd left home with two), backpack, or *Blues Clues* jukebox. No doubt he'd destroyed his shirts. But where was everything else?

A day of dejection ensued. He'd been miserable. Had we been selfish?

We'd now visited nine schools. Every nearby place had significant flaws, and the distant schools either had no openings or didn't want Cam. We honestly didn't believe we were being too choosy, unconsciously picking nits to sabotage the search.

But two months into our odyssey, we felt no further along than we'd been in May. It was hard not to feel discouraged. For the next several days, I asked myself over and over whether we were making the right decision. Just as troubling was another question that I couldn't quash: what if only Shelter Beach accepted him? When I'd described the place to Les, I'd declared, "I'd rather keep him home than send him there."

It was looking like I might get my wish.

Chapter 19

Returns

> . . . the end of all our exploring
> Will be to arrive where we started
> And know the place for the first time.
> —T. S. Eliot, "Little Gidding"

The Twilight Zone

On Cam's twelfth birthday I happened to watch "It's a *Good* Life," a chilling *Twilight Zone* episode about a boy named Anthony who uses supernatural powers to turn adults into his slaves. Imperial little Anthony dictates what to play on the piano, what TV shows to watch, what and when to eat; he even summons a deadly midsummer snowstorm. Anyone who fails to cater to his whims gets "wished away to the cornfield" and ceases to exist. With frozen smiles glued to their faces, the adults watch Anthony's TV show—a dinosaur battle—and simper, "That was real good! . . . It was much better than the old television."

One poor soul named Dan can take no more: it's *his* birthday, and he isn't even allowed to listen to his new Perry Como record! After getting drunk, he points menacingly at Anthony's parents: "You! You had him!"

Anthony fixes the man with a demonic glower. "You're a *bad* man," he declares, and turns Dan into a jack-in-the-box. Afterward, Anthony's father assures him, "It's *good* what you done to Dan. It's *real* good."

The show seemed all too familiar. Didn't Les and I also watch the same childish TV programs day in and day out, cater to our son's musical choices, and ply him with treats? Hadn't our son also sent us places we'd never wished to go? Didn't our house also seem frozen in time, as Cam spent his birthday doing the same things he had done every day for five, six, seven years?

We didn't need Rod Serling to break the news; it was obvious where we lived.

One thing *was* different about this birthday: it might be the last one our Yankee Doodle dandy spent at home. Though years of disappointment had taught us to scale down birthday celebrations, for some reason this year Cam expected something extraordinary. The previous day we'd told him there might be a party at school. He didn't see the cupcakes we'd packed and neither of us mentioned the event, but as he prepared for school he spontaneously sang "Happy Birthday." The hopeful parents in us wanted to believe he knew the calendar and remembered the date of his birthday; the more sensible part figured someone at school had mentioned it.

Still, we didn't make much of the day, other than taking him to the bakery to choose a cake. Though he couldn't tell time, he'd enjoyed wearing Les's sports watch that summer, so we bought him a colorful cheap watch. Recalling last year's limited success, we also tried to interest him in *The Wizard of Oz*.

When the Munchkins sang "Ding, Dong, the witch is dead," Cam briefly perked up, but soon his requests for "Poppins" grew insistent. Even after we put the *Poppins* tape in, he couldn't settle down. Finally, amidst a flurry of angry gibberish, an intelligible word emerged—"presents." He had been cruelly denied a real birthday.

I said to Les, "Well, he's right. We didn't do much to celebrate. We're treating him like a dog instead of a kid." She scoffed but still scurried out to buy more presents.

When she returned, she asked, "If you'd told your parents on your birthday, 'I want more presents,' would they have dashed out to buy you something else?" I laughed sarcastically. Were we overindulging him?

Cam's response answered the question. He avidly played with his new phone—which spoke the number, counted the rings, played tunes—then ran through the house, bounced on his tramp, and shouted, "Eeeehhh! Ha, ha, ha, ha! Hee, hee, hee!" It was the greatest invention in the history of technology. We had to pry it from his fingers to get him to sleep.

His joy was no greater than ours. Maybe we were guilt-ridden dupes. But what did that matter next to our son's delight?

We agreed: it was *good* that we'd bought him more presents.

Escape Clause

The birthday was the first of many returns that July, as we awaited the results of school visits and planned return trips. Wallbrook had requested a second interview, but we'd already made up our minds to reject the school and decided that emphasizing Cam's aggression would guarantee that they'd return the favor. We needed them to reject us, because otherwise the state might force Cam to go somewhere unsuitable.

After we greeted the admissions officer, Cam touched every object in the room, then rocked boisterously in a Naugahyde chair. We couldn't conduct an interview with him there, so I led him to a room across the hall while Les continued.

A red-haired teenager entered, accompanied by a short black man. The boy opened a bag of corn chips, dumped them on the floor, swept them into a pile and crushed them before putting the crumbs into his mouth.

"Does he want a snack?" the man asked me about Cam, his words lengthened by an African lilt. "He is a very special guest, so he may have a juice. Would he like corn chips?"

"That'd be great. Thanks."

Other kids wandered in to collect their backpacks and get ready for the buses. The noise prompted a volley of belches from Cam, then loud, guttural shouts. Amid this din, a chubby boy of about thirteen entered, jammed his fingers into his ears, and sat on the pillows stacked in the corner, talking to himself. Soon he started to growl and thrash.

The African man approached me and spoke, but the racket drowned out his words.

I stared blankly at him.

"He becomes *a*ggressive," he clarified, accenting the first syllable.

"So does my son," I replied. Then I got the message: we could have a brawl on our hands. We discreetly made our exit.

Cam entertained himself for fifteen minutes by swinging—high, higher, then so high that his legs poked above the crossbar. I joined him in a nearby swing until I began to feel queasy.

When most of the kids had departed, we returned to the conference room. The interview had gone well: Les had made it plain that we hadn't been impressed by Wallbrook at our first visit. "We've had some staffing problems," the lady had admitted. They were troubled by Cam's recent outbursts on the bus: every student here rode a bus to and from the residences daily.

"Yes," Les had said, "those were very scary. They even had to add another matron just for Cam. But he's always had problems on the bus, going back to when he was five. They worry us too, because something terrible could happen."

Both women knew what was going on: we'd given Wallbrook an escape clause, and they were going to grab it. As soon as Les conveyed our message, the lady couldn't get rid of her fast enough. "I thought she was going to start shoving me in the back," she told me.

On the way home we stopped for milkshakes at Arby's. Cam had never drunk one before, but he enjoyed the first half before dumping the remainder into the armrest. The rest of the trip was less smooth than the shake. First we got caught in the usual DC beltway gridlock. As we crept along, Cam said, "Potty."

There was no way I was going to exit and then try to reenter the parking lot that was I-495. "We can't stop, buddy. Go ahead and go potty in your pants. It's okay this time."

Cam grumbled but didn't kick. A few minutes later, he repeated, "Potty," this time in an agitated voice.

"We probably better get off before he starts a kickfest," I suggested. "Can he just go in a parking lot or something?"

"He did it on the way back from camp," Les answered, "so I don't see why not."

We stayed on the exit ramp for what seemed like an hour, every second expecting Cam to start planting kicks at our shoulders, before spotting a bank parking lot. I careened around a sharp corner and screeched to a halt, tires straddling the yellow lines. Les thrust open the door, unlatched Cam's seatbelt, and helped him pull down his pants.

"Go ahead and go potty, sweetie. It's okay here."

He stood for a minute, looking confused. Then a stream of creamy liquid spewed from his mouth. Then another. Vanilla milkshake spattered Leslie's tan pumps.

We wrapped our brave boy in his favorite blanket and sped away. We'd never before seen him get carsick, but it seemed fitting. As we neared home Les said what we were both thinking: "I guess Cam made his statement about Wallbrook!"

Jeopardy

The next Tuesday Cam's school report listed ninety-five aggressions. Wednesday was the day of his interview at Three Sisters. We beseeched the universal powers: please let him behave!

Maybe somebody heard us, because Cam was an angel. He played with his toy phone and smiled genially at everyone while Carla, the admissions specialist, and Jane Crockett, the slender, blonde speech pathologist, discussed him with us. Aware that he was the center of attention, Cam gave his best performance.

I asked him his name, where he lived, his age—questions he'd learned to answer in our functional language drill. When he didn't respond, my face reddened. On the third try, he finally answered.

"Cam, where do you live?"

"Baaalmore."

"What's your address?"

"Tweebrook."

"How old are you?"

"Eeeeh. Hah! Lu-lu-lu." He spun the chair around.

"Cam. How old are you?" Come on, buddy, this is why we practiced all those years!

He looked down.

"Cameron, how old are you?" Les asked.

"Leben twelve."

"He still thinks he's eleven," I explained.

"Well, it's so new!" sympathized Carla. I didn't mention the months of drilling needed to replace "ten" with "'leben."

They asked about the bus incidents. "How long has that been going on?"

"We had one serious incident at the end of the school year. But he's been riding the bus since he was four," I said, "and in those eight years there've been maybe two incidents."

"It's quite a major part of their clinical report."

"They're exaggerating," Les said. She didn't mention that we'd used the incident to scare off other schools.

Crockett asked why Cam didn't have a communication device available during the session shown on the video.

"That's a darn good question, isn't it?" I said. "That's just one of many reasons we're leaving that school." It had taken three years of our nagging to get Cam a voice output device, and then nobody knew how to use it. But this woman knew exactly how to use one. For the first time in weeks I remembered that we weren't just looking for a *different* school for Cam; we were looking for a *better* school. All at once my attitude underwent a sea change. This didn't mean we were giving up on Cam. It meant we *weren't* giving up on him!

As if on cue, Crockett asked, "What are your hopes for Cameron?" I looked at Les for help. Her brown eyes brimmed with tears.

I cleared my throat. "We want him to be happy. We want to find a place where he'll succeed and thrive. He needs more structure than we can give him. We need a school that will accept him as he is but also help him do better." I stopped. There was so much to say, so many words, none of them adequate.

Carla and Jane also had tears in their eyes.

Meanwhile, Cam played with his phone, spun, jumped, and clapped. Did he realize we were looking for a new place for him to live?

At the end of the interview, Jane said, "He has lots of potential." We hadn't heard *that* in quite awhile! They saw something in his bright eyes and boundless energy.

At last we took a walk—Cam holding my hand, then flinging it away, stopping, running, stopping, running—through the school. We met the sister in charge of what would be Cam's dorm, and watched students moving from classes to the dorms. Most seemed more capable and more focused than our son. Would he rise to their level?

Throughout the tour, Cam's toy phone kept ringing; at each ring the staff members looked around, then smiled at us. It almost seemed someone were trying to send a message. Then the boy himself sent one.

"Coke!"

Please, I thought, let us find one before he blows up! We found the vending machines, but when Les put a Coke in front of him, he "no, okayed" it; he wanted to leave. As Les finished up with Carla, I sat tensely beside Cam, who sprawled restlessly on the couch. Miraculously, he kept his cool until we left.

We were thoughtful on the rainy drive home. Three Sisters was close enough to visit frequently. The staff cared about the kids and already had plans for our son. But we'd seen only a couple of other autistic students. Would this regimented environment help him stay calm? Or would he turn the place upside down? We agreed it was easily the best of the Maryland schools, but it was scarcely a perfect fit: Cam seemed too active, too *autistic* for them.

We also worried about the long breaks in June and August. We'd have no home program in place and we'd all struggle to adjust. Carla had told us that many students went to camp on breaks. But Camp Wonder was out of the picture. Was this drawback serious enough to eliminate them? In any case, the whole discussion seemed moot, for neither of us believed they'd accept him.

Skip, Skip, Skip

By July 20, more returns were flowing in. Wallbrook (to our relief) rejected Cam. Garden Grove needed a referral from our school district, but it wasn't on Baltimore County's list of approved schools, which meant we'd have to be rejected by all Maryland schools before the county could even begin to consider them. It was out of the running. But Shelter Beach wanted Cam. If no other Maryland school accepted him, we'd have to go to court and prove it was inappropriate before we could get an out-of-state placement.

That day we also heard from BenPenn, a well-regarded facility not far away. It immediately became a leading candidate.

You know the first four bars of "Skip to My Lou?" Me too: in fact, I'll never forget them. The version on Cam's keyboard features a drum intro, then the melody on piano: "Dum, dum, dum-dah-dah-doo, do-do-do-do dah *dah* dah!" After a drum roll and cymbal crash, a motherly voice intones, "Hi! Let's play!" Not once on the two-hours-plus drive to BenPenn did Cam press the button for "Bingo" or "John Jacob Jingleheimer Schmidt." No: we skipped until we could skip no more.

But once we arrived, Cam wouldn't skip; he wouldn't even budge from the back seat, despite offers of a Coke and snack. When we finally coaxed him from the car, he walked twenty feet and went on a sit-down strike. I hunted for the admissions officer while Les stayed with Cam.

I wandered around the building—a converted country mansion, complete with winding staircase and gingerbread porch—until I met a pleasant-looking woman named Catalina Gomez. She helped cajole Cam into the building, and a few minutes later we sat around a shiny oval table with a nurse and the director of admissions, Paul McCallum, a professorial man with a graying beard and a slight British accent. Meanwhile, Cam denuded a boxwood twig he'd brought with him, tore apart a string, and roved the room emptying coffee cups onto the floor. Les or I jumped up every fifteen seconds to prevent him from shredding their pothos plant.

"What kinds of things does Cameron like to do?" the nurse asked.

"You're looking at it," Les answered sardonically. Then she smiled, adding that he also liked music and swimming.

After some talk about communication systems, I recounted our attempts to teach Cam to read, write, and speak. "We've worked and worked but his abilities are still very limited. The behaviors get in the way. He understands a lot, and tries hard to talk, but often can't recall the word. Then he gets frustrated and acts up."

As I finished the sentence, Cam gave a loud whine of distress. His downturned mouth and tearful eyes illustrated his frustration much better than my outline. As I patted his arm, I felt my eyes fill up. "But you really try, son, we know you do." McCallum had taken in my summary with noncommittal "uh-hms," but his eyebrows went up during this last exchange.

In the on-campus group home, a supervisor described activities, schedules, behavioral protocols. A tall teenage resident helped a female staff member do some baking; two other residents placidly watched a video. The house was clean, orderly, and businesslike; picture schedules covered the walls. I was impressed.

McCallum then led me to back to the school, down two flights of stairs, and around a corner to the basement, where the classroom for kids with "challenging behaviors" was located. A young teacher named Mike was compiling data from the day.

I asked him, "Have you dealt with a lot of aggression? Cameron can get very wild. He sometimes hits, bites, and pulls hair."

Mike smiled slightly. One of his students, he told me, was a big seventeen-year-old whose brain injury had made him subject to explosive outbursts. He pointed to a large hole in the wall the young man had created with his fist.

"For the first two weeks, we had to alternate fifteen-minute shifts with him, so the staff didn't get burned out or hurt." He paused. "But now he works by himself, sits quietly between breaks and hasn't had a tantrum for months." With another smile, he glanced up at me. "So I doubt Cam could throw anything at us that we haven't seen before."

I had to laugh. "You make a strong case!"

McCallum and Gomez assured us that they were interested in Cam. A team would discuss him and get back to me within the week.

But when I called a few days later, they sang a different tune. McCallum turned cagey, telling me they'd just hired a new autism specialist who planned a slew of ambitious projects. "We are likely to remain in a holding pattern for a few months until we determine what resources—both human and financial—we'll need to carry them out."

"Oh. Where does this put Cameron? Does he have any chance for acceptance at BenPenn?"

"We remain quite interested in Cameron," he said. "But we've recently admitted several students who require a good deal of behavioral support. We will have to evaluate whether we can adequately serve his needs, given the requirements of this cohort of new students."

What was he was trying to tell me? He continued. "You see, we try to keep a balance in our population."

I got it. "You can't take on too many 'lower-functioning' students at one time?"

"Well, yes, that's about right. You see, these students are very staff intensive. So it may be that the timing is not quite right."

It was a tactful brush off. Consumed with disappointment, I hung up the phone. BenPenn had seemed the best fit so far.

We'd lost our partner. What would we do?

Sunrise

With the horizon obscured by clouds of doubt and fear, our twilight zone was darker than ever. Then suddenly the sun broke through: Three Sisters called to tell us they had accepted Cameron into their program. They were careful to inform us of their ten-day trial period: if they decided that they couldn't work with him or he couldn't adjust, they could send him back. Nevertheless, when

Les got home, we hugged, kissed, and leaped around the kitchen. Clearly they'd seen *something* in our son.

Over the previous two months, I'd stayed busy so as not to dwell on what all these trips and preparations meant. I hadn't believed that any Maryland school would accept Cam. My crystal ball, frosted over by years of disappointment, had told me that come fall nothing would have changed, except that we could reassure ourselves we'd done everything possible. The failure would be the county's, the schools', autism's—anyone's but ours.

But now the fateful moment had arrived. I knew the right thing to do, knew that for our family to survive and for Cameron to thrive, we had to send him to a residential school. Yet the day after Three Sisters broke their news, all the sadness, misgivings, and guilt I'd been suppressing came surging back. The twilight zone suddenly seemed a comfortable place to dwell.

Les was irritated. "I don't know what to say to you. After three months of looking for a school you suddenly have cold feet! Think about what's best for Buddy!"

I heard her words, but didn't feel them. What finally showed me the light was a feature article in the Baltimore *Sun* about the Goodmans, whose son Mitchell had been in Cam's class for several years.

The reporter was obsessed with Mitchell's behaviors. There were plenty to document: he walked on his tiptoes, rarely made eye contact, didn't talk, and once had broken his mother's coffee cup and stomped on it, severely gashing his foot. Five adults had had to hold him while he got stitches. He bit himself so frequently that he had to wear thick gloves and arm guards.

The lead photo displayed a portrait of this autist: Mitchell kneeling, hands splayed out against a large window, pushing his face against the pane as if trying to break through. The story starkly depicted the other inmates: a mother so sleep-deprived and anxious that she lost her train of thought in the middle of sentences; a father whose hyperanimated garrulity betrayed a desperate need for others to share his pain. Yet when the reporter asked about finding Mitchell a different place to live, the mother recoiled; she couldn't bear the thought. And instead of planning for the immediate future, the father fantasized about building a group home for Mitchell as an adult.

I understood them: better to maintain what's familiar, no matter how dreadful, than try something different. But these folks were seriously in denial. Couldn't they see how crazy their lives were?

Then, suddenly, I realized I was reading about myself. I too was afraid to throw off the blinders of guilt and exhaustion and take a clear-eyed look at the road ahead. All at once my ambivalence vanished. We'd come too far to turn back now. We had to help Cam escape before the prison doors slammed shut for good.

We called Carla at Three Sisters and told her we were surprised at her news.

"I'm surprised you're surprised. The team was pretty much unanimous." We felt reassured. But now it was our turn to leave somebody hanging: before accepting their offer, we'd proceed with the planned visit to Bright Spirit. If that didn't change our minds, we'd agree to the placement at Three Sisters. We told Carla we needed a few days to think about it.

The Outer Limits

I slept badly the night before my trip to Kansas. Every half hour I heard Cam shout and roll around, and was already awake when the alarm went off at 5:40.

The journey—a three-hour flight to Kansas City followed by three more hours of driving through the hot, windswept prairie—was a marathon, but somehow I arrived twenty minutes early. While waiting, I gazed out the window at the sparkling campus—brand new buildings, green lawns and trees (a little droopy in the sweltering weather), glittering pond—and felt the school was aptly named. A glow seemed to surround the place, as if it weren't Kansas but Oz or Brigadoon. I had the unsettling sense that if I opened a hidden door I'd see the machine that had generated it all and watch the whole gleaming vista vanish in a puff of smoke.

Tara, the youthful, bubbly admissions officer, embodied the school's image, as did the executive vice president, a fleshy man with elaborately brushed hair who exuded the polished aura of one accustomed to giving fund-raising speeches. Some of their canned phrases ("we don't believe in maintenance," "we value parental input") invaded our conversation, as he explained their mission to educate kids that other schools wouldn't take. That meant every student had a "para"—a one-on-one paraprofessional aide. He seemed personable and dedicated, though when I elaborated on Cam's quirks and habits, I caught him sneaking peeks at his watch.

The educational director, a thin, dark man in his forties, showed me several classrooms where kids were hard at work with "paras." Bright Spirit's rooms were much bigger and airier than those of any other school I'd seen; the staff took constant data. I watched a wide-mouthed girl devour Froot Loops as the director proudly told of their success with aggressive students.

The kids in Cam's prospective class were on a trip to a botanical garden. "Cam would love that," I told the teacher. "He could strip those rare plants down to twigs in minutes."

She looked at me quizzically. "Well, maybe we'd give him something else to do."

Next was the medical department. As Head Nurse Janie, a woman with the brisk, no-nonsense demeanor of an office manager, rolled out her set speech about doctors and drugs, students stopped by for afternoon meds.

A dark-haired teenager strode in and announced, "You know what? I caught . . . a big . . . fish. In the newspaper." The phrases emerged laboriously, each word packed with pent-up effort.

"That's great, Tim," Tara said. She looked at me and grinned, pleased but faintly embarrassed. What was there to be embarrassed about? My child could barely talk at all. Then Tim told us about the fish again. Then again. And then again, each time using the same words in the same order. He would have kept going, but Janie interrupted to suggest that he go back to class. As he was leaving, he told us he'd gone to a hockey game with his dad.

"Oh, you mean at Christmas?" Nurse Janie said. It seemed like only yesterday to him.

"My dad said . . . I could play for the Rivermen!"

Tim stood at least 5' 10" and probably had to shave every day, yet had the social awareness of a four-year-old. But to me he was a success story. I nursed a pang of envy.

It was nearing 4 p.m., and the lack of sleep was catching up with me. The speech path, a loquacious redhead with a husky voice, may have sensed my flagging attention, for she gave me a lot more information than I needed, recalling in great detail the many "kiddos" she'd treated in her eleven years. I even learned that she'd once been a dental hygienist.

Still, I was impressed by her *functional* approach to language. "You put pictures in front of a kiddo all day and say, 'show me apple.' After a few times he's thinking, 'Would you knock it off, lady? I know what an apple is, but I don't feel like doing this dumb drill.'"

Cam's speech pathologists had repeated the same drills for years and then complained that he was "noncompliant." These folks *did* seem to have brighter ideas.

At the group home (right on campus), the director, a lively African American woman named Sheila, eagerly showed me the place. Every kid had his or her own room, and Cam's was already picked out. But one young man spent the duration of my forty-five-minute visit sitting on the floor and spinning a piece of yarn. Another resident, a quiet little guy in a helmet, paced nervously around the house. Were their school districts getting their money's worth?

Enter Mickey, a muscular young man who shoved his face two inches from mine and gleefully flipped a straw he clutched in his fist. He said hello by popping air bubbles inside his cheeks and spraying my chin with saliva. Chuckling at his private joke, he placed his hand on my throat and stared disconcertingly into my eyes.

His para pulled hard at his hand. "Mickey, you have to ask to touch."

"Oh, it's okay," I assured her. Would he try this with Cam?

Suddenly we heard a loud clunk. The helmeted boy had pitched to the floor and landed on his head; he was having a seizure. Staff members gathered around, taking his pulse and talking to him. Sheila blandly informed me that if they couldn't rouse him within a minute they'd inject him with antiseizure medicine. I tried not to look rattled.

When they were sure he was okay, Sheila asked me, "What does Cameron like to do?" I stifled the urge to say, "Oh, tear clothes, strip tree branches, wreck furniture. You know, the usual," and mentioned music, videos, push-button toys. Then I thought, "What the hell, why not prepare them for the worst?" and launched into a detailed account of his aggression, disruptions, and property destruction.

Sheila's smile faded. "He sounds interesting," she said. The old Chinese curse again.

That evening the ed director, school psychologist, Tara, and Joseph Woodward, the admissions officer I'd met in June, took me to dinner at a Tex-Mex restaurant. They assured me they were looking forward to meeting Cam when (they seemed certain) he enrolled in September. Only once did their veneer crack: when Woodward noted in passing that Cam was "more involved" (that is, more severely disabled) than Bobby, a teenager from Cam's school now at Bright Spirit. At fourteen, Bobby was not even toilet trained. I must have made a face, for the psychologist quickly added that Cam was considered more "involved" because of his aggression. I remembered Woodward's comments about the pacifier. What else were they saying when I wasn't around?

It was hard not to be flattered by the red-carpet treatment, and I spent the drive back to Kansas City enveloped in a warm glow. The place seemed like paradise. But as the hours passed, the aura dimmed. I felt as if I were emerging from a hypnotic state, and recalled an old TV show—I think it was *The Outer Limits*—in which aliens welcome earthlings to their planet by giving them a tour of the beautiful village where they'll live. Once the visitors settle in, they learn that the village is a giant trap enticing them into becoming lab animals for a race of monstrous aliens. Of course, no such sinister design was operating here. Yet I wondered if Bright Spirit worked so hard to enchant parents so we wouldn't notice the man behind the curtain. For they had one insuperable problem no smoke and mirrors could disguise—location. Their wizardry couldn't hide the fact that they *were* in Kansas.

I'd left home at 6 a.m. and arrived at the school at 1 p.m. their time. That included no delays in the airport or on the tarmac. How would we even get Cameron here? There was no way he could take a commercial flight, and what was the alternative? Two or three torturous days in the car? Chartering a plane? None of these options seemed remotely feasible.

Later I realized that location wasn't even the real problem. It was this: if we sent Cam to Bright Spirit, we'd be closing the door and turning out the lights on our life with him. The school had a week-long June break and an optional break at the holidays, which meant we'd see our son for at most two weeks a year. Sure, we could visit him occasionally, but the marathon I'd just completed wasn't one we could repeat often. We weren't ready to write Cam out of our lives so completely.

After all the preparations, trips, agonized discussions, the choice turned out to be easy. Two days after I returned from Kansas, we accepted Three Sisters' offer.

Great Expectations

Our odyssey had ended. Three Sisters was our fate. Yet in some ways we remained in the twilight zone. Though we vowed to do everything to make sure they didn't send Cam back for a refund after the ten-day trial period, we still doubted he'd make it.

I felt blue, but Les maintained *her* bright spirit: "Buddy is going off to find his way in the world," she said. She jabbed her right fist into her left palm. "This is his chance to *make* something of himself!"

She was right: we had to believe that our little Pip had great expectations. We had to believe the new school would let us celebrate a new independence day. We had to believe that our best gift to Cam would be this chance for a re-birthday.

Chapter 20

Nosology

How poor are they that have not patience!
What wound ever did heal but by degrees?
—Shakespeare, *Othello*

Look with Thine Ears

In early July 2001, Dr. Robert Lauschen, a wiry, bearded psychiatrist with a piercing gaze, listened intently to our stories of life with Cam. He pointed out that our narratives didn't jibe, and that my story about seeking a residential placement—a story about failure, as he put it—didn't fit the facts.

He told us we were suffering from post-traumatic stress disorder, compounded by exhaustion and resentment. After working long hours at her stressful job, Leslie came home to a second, equally stressful shift. She believed I calculated the time I spent with Cam and insinuated that she owed me. I denied it but admitted to feeling resentment at having to do so much by myself. I keep hammering even after the nail is bent. I call this trait tenacity; my wife calls it obstinacy. Whatever you call it, it had made me refuse help even when I could no longer handle Cam's autism.

Dr. Lauschen helped us see two other facts: Les was inclined to be overprotective and unstinting; and I was filled with rage. These facts collided during

Cam's outbursts: I furiously confronted him; Les criticized me and "interfered" (my term), further enraging me and frightening Cam. She insisted that she was protecting him from me. But what was I doing? Was I protecting Les from Cam, punishing Cam, or just defending myself from the unpredictable creature who occupied our house?

The doctor warned that this pattern was dangerous and urged us to change it "before someone ends up in prison." My mouth dropped open: prison? Then I recalled the fury I'd felt during one recent confrontation with Cam and gulped: yes, I'd been angry enough to hurt someone.

He suggested that this pattern derived partly from our childhoods: Les's as an oldest sibling charged with supervising three younger brothers; mine as the son of a heavy-drinking father. She had transformed me into the unrelenting parent and Cam into the siblings whose needs were never satisfied. I had turned Cam into the sometimes belligerent, sometimes maudlin father who had made me feel powerless.

The doctor talked a lot about our "narratives." If you can alter the stories you tell yourself and become more self-conscious about the patterns that produce these battles, he told us, you can change the outcome.

I understood that I'd been viewing the world through distorted lenses. I needed to see and hear Cam, Leslie, and myself more clearly. Would this therapy make Cam less aggressive? No. Would it help him verbalize his fears and anxieties? No. The doctor was right: we felt helpless. But our feelings of helplessness were nothing compared to Cam's.

Cam could hardly do talk therapy; his psychiatrist's main job was to monitor his medication. But Cam hated visiting Dr. Rodriguez—hated the waiting, hated listening to us talk about him. So I tried to make our mid-July visit sound like an adventure. Since Les was meeting us there, I said, "Cam, let's get in the car and go see Mommy!"

He refused to put on his pants and then ran away, but eventually got into the car. About five minutes from the doctor's office, he began to shout the now-dreaded word "Coke," and by the time we rolled into the parking lot, he was thumping my shoulder with his foot. I recalled Dr. Lauschen's advice: catch yourself before you react instinctively. So instead of shouting and pushing Cam's foot, I just dodged and thought about a tough piece I was learning on the sax. The strategy worked: I kept my temper and coaxed Cam out of the car without escalating the conflict.

Twenty-five minutes passed before we were shown into Dr. Rodriguez's tiny, cluttered office.

"Well, how are we doing?" she asked.

"Better," we agreed.

"Let's see your arms." We held out our arms like kids being checked for grime. "Parents are too tolerant," she said. "But the arms don't lie." I had only the fading bite scar; Les's marks had grown faint. As we discussed drugs and hospitals, Cam quietly shredded a shoe lace and rocked in his chair. What did he think when we described his aggression? What did he make of the talk about side effects? Sure, he heard us; but did he *hear* us?

Cam's ears became important in another way soon after, when he jammed a wad of string into his left ear. This was an old, bad habit we'd thought was gone forever.

You can't just poke tweezers into an ear as you might a drain, and the job gets even trickier when the patient won't sit still. That was the case with Cam, who flinched and twitched as soon as he spied the tweezers. The more we tried to hold him, the more nervous he became, and if Les raised her voice he jumped up and fled. He knew he was supposed to be still but couldn't control his instinctive recoil. If I tried to hold him down, he'd roll around like a pinned wrestler. Les tried talking to him quietly. It was working: as she approached with the Q-tip, he held his head still, still, still . . . until she touched his ear. Then he jerked away, squealing, "Eee-dee-dee-dee!"

This frustrating ritual continued for a good half-hour: time after time she calmly approached him and brought the tweezers or Q-tip closer and closer, only to have Cam lurch away just when she had touched the embedded string. Twenty tries brought no results.

For once Les was the one who lost her temper. Throwing her hands into the air, she shouted, "Hold still! Oh! I just want to kill him! Just fucking hold still, will you?"

"Yelling at him won't help."

"Oh shut up! If you think you can do any better, go ahead and try."

"Calm down. We'll figure something out." I tried to hold Cam's head still.

"Don't tell me to calm down! And don't hold his head, you're making it worse!"

A look of shock passed over Cam's face. Mommy never screamed like this.

We counted to twenty while Les stuck a flashlight into her mouth, shined it into his ear and tried to pluck out the string. Several times she got the tweezers into the opening of his ear canal, only to be defeated again by a last-second flinch. By now, Cam was beating his chest in fear, and his parents were bellowing at each other.

"Oh!" Les finally said in a choked voice, "I have to go the bedroom or I'm going to hit somebody!"

When she returned, I said, "We could go to a doctor, but how is a doctor going to get it out if he won't hold still?"

"Oh, don't start that Eeyore crap. They've done this before, so I'm sure they have methods."

"Yeah, like what? If he won't hold still for us, what makes you think he'll do it for them?" I raised my eyes to the ceiling. "God! Why won't he just hold still?"

"Because he doesn't have a brain. God damn it! I hate this life! I want to throttle my own kid. Jesus! He doesn't even have enough sense to hold his head still! He has the IQ of a newt!"

Her shoulders slumped.

"Night after night after night we just wait for the little tyrant to fall asleep. Then I'm too tired to do anything. This is hell, a living hell."

I couldn't argue. But I too was shocked at Leslie's rage. It was as if between us we carried a set quantity of anger, and when I didn't show it, she had to.

Several minutes of silence passed as we sat despondently on the sofa. Then I grabbed the flashlight and tweezers, knelt by Cam's bed and showed him the light.

"Daddy's just going to look in your ear. No tweezers. Do you want to hold the light?"

Cam took the flashlight and tried to shine it into his ear.

"Good job, Cam. Thanks for helping Daddy." I let him do it three or four more times. "Now, can you hold the light while Daddy looks? Good. Okay, now hold still."

As soon as I picked up the tweezers, he dropped the light and began to rock and roll, repeating, "Ho'd till, ho'd till."

"That's right, hold still, son." But he couldn't hold still.

Eventually I got a glimpse into his ears. I couldn't see anything.

A few minutes later Cam ventured out, casting wary glances around. Soon he was sitting next to Les on the couch, nuzzling and kissing her cheek.

"IQ of a newt, eh?"

"Mommy never gets that mad," she said, her brown eyes shining.

Opposable

A week later, Cam's therapist, Jim, returned from their ride with a horror story. On the way to 7–11, Cam had start grabbing and kicking him. In Jim's sports car there was nowhere to hide, so he'd had to fend off Cam's blows for several minutes.

I'd asked him why he didn't just get out of the car.

"My car is so full of junk that I was afraid he'd break something or hurt himself."

The excuse seemed dubious, but I really couldn't blame him: I knew better than anyone how hard it is to think straight at such moments. Jim had brought

Cam to his own house, let him go potty, and given him some crackers. He'd gradually calmed down.

Cam was still cranky after Jim left, and at dinner I noticed that he was holding his spoon with his third and fourth fingers instead of his index finger and thumb. We examined his hand: his thumb was swollen and bruised at the bottom joint.

"Do you think it's broken?" Les asked.

"Let's see if he can move it. Cam, can you move your thumb like this?" I made the thumbs-up gesture, then realized the absurdity of the request: despite hundreds of hours of occupational therapy, Cam couldn't make a thumbs-up on command even when his hand was uninjured. We diagnosed a sprain, gave him two Motrin, and within a half hour he cheered up.

We didn't. How *had* Cam hurt his thumb? I knew I hadn't done it. Had Jim accidentally—or, God forbid, intentionally—injured Cam's thumb during the episode in the car?

"I've never trusted that Jim," said Les.

"Oh, come on. He's been working with Cam for months, and I've been here almost every time. He likes Cam and does really well with him. But he could have twisted it just trying to protect himself."

"Or he could've lost his temper. It's my worst fear—somebody's going to hurt him and he can't tell us!"

How would we know if Cam were molested or hurt at his new, faraway school? To resist fighting back when our aggressive twelve-year-old slapped or bit you required superhuman self-control. We were his parents and *we* wanted to hurt him sometimes. Just one momentary impulse and Cam could be injured. Or . . . worse.

We tried not to think about it. But the fears didn't dissolve.

I feigned nonchalance as we found a seat in the pediatricians' waiting room; Cam's "Skip to My Lou" keyboard seemed overbearingly loud. In the exam room, he dumped his Coke into the sink and ran water at full blast into the cup. Soon water was streaming over the sides of the sink and splashing onto the floor. I couldn't move: what the hell, at least he was occupied. When the puddle got large, I took away the cup and cleaned up with a paper towel. Would the doctor never come?

A Polish woman, Dr. Brodsky, had taken over Dr. Archer's practice when he'd retired. Although she resembled a grade-school principal—stern face, iron gray hair, sensible shoes—her sweet manner always won Cam's cooperation.

She examined his thumb and recommended an X-ray. Then she let Cam touch and examine the otoscope light; he actually let her peer into his ear canal for a few seconds. She stroked his arm. "You're such a good boy," she said, her Polish accent coloring her words.

"I don't see anything in de ear, and I was able to see de tympanic membrane."

"Could it still be in there?"

"Yes, it might be out of sight. If you see a discharge, or he starts favoring his ear, then you need to call me."

"What happens then?"

"We'll have to hold him down and take it out."

"That ought to be fun."

For the X-ray, we went to St. Giles—the hospital where Cam had been born twelve years earlier—but I was too anxious to savor any ironies. On the elevator, I placed myself between Cam and the four adults sharing the car, pretending I wasn't poised on the balls of my feet, prepared to spring into action at his slightest movement.

When we reached the radiology waiting room, I left Cam in a chair while the receptionist quizzed me about medical history and insurance. A well-meaning secretary brought a large box of Legos that Cam immediately dumped onto the floor and then ignored; he was far more interested in plucking an artificial daisy. An elderly man and woman gawked unabashedly at Cam's attempts to tear apart the flower.

I heard the lady say, "Doesn't it break your heart?" The man's face wore the now-familiar blend of fascination, pity, and thin-lipped judgment. I could almost hear his thoughts: "That kid just needs a good spanking!"

I planted myself between Cam and the daisy. He pinched my arm until it bled. I clenched my teeth and tried to keep my eyes wide and blank while whispering, "Cam. Stop pinching my arm. Stop it!" He twisted my pinkie instead. Sweat stood out on my forehead. Well, I reasoned, if he breaks my finger at least I can get it X-rayed right away.

At last we were called into the X-ray room. I explained Cam's disability briefly to the technician, who smiled and asked him to put his right hand on the table so we could take a picture of it. Cam promptly placed his left hand on the table.

"Other hand, Cameron," she said.

He put both hands on the table.

Eventually we got pictures of his thumb, but Cam had moved so much that the second one came out blurry and we had to take another. While we waited for them to be developed, my son squirmed, bounced on the chair, and sprawled over the X-ray table, his feet pushing against my shoulder. I suddenly realized that I'd forgotten to give him his afternoon pill. No wonder he was so agitated. But who knew this was going to take so long?

The technician finally returned. As Cam twisted my fingers into pretzels, I looked over the X-rays and tried to converse with her. We saw no sign of a broken bone but had to wait for a doctor to confirm our conclusion.

More waiting: Cam rolled around on the table. Any second now I was going to burst into a howl. Just in time, the technician returned: the doctor had confirmed that there was no fracture.

Cam's thumb was intact, but my nerves were torn into tiny pieces.

Ecce Homo

Cam's thumb healed and he stopped pulling at his ear. After all the poking and prodding, the traumatic visits to the doctor, the shouting and fear, most kids would never again shove anything into an orifice. Most kids. But over the years Cam had crammed a variety of items—strings, seeds, rice kernels, pieces of plastic—into his ears and nose. They'd always come back out, either after an agonizing session with the tweezers like the one described above or after a violent bout of sneezing.

We speculated that he liked the feeling of sneezing, that there was something satisfying about the tickle and violent expulsion. Perhaps he didn't think beyond, "Gee, that thing will fit right up my nose!" Or if he did consider consequences, they mattered less than the immediate sensual gratification. Incidents like these reminded us of the real meaning of cognitive impairment: an inability to foresee effects or learn from experience.

More painful was the recognition that he did these things because he was bored. He was learning nothing at school; it was becoming too risky to take him into public places; he'd never learned to play and rejected new experiences. The objects in Cam's nose and ears were symbols of our entrapment in autism's vicious circle and of why we needed a way out.

Sunday, July 29, was a quiet day. Les went to her office for a couple of hours while I watched a ball game in the den and let Cam entertain himself. Bad move. Before long I heard the convulsive sneezing that meant Cam had stuffed something up his nose.

I looked into his left nostril. I could just make out a piece of white plastic, maybe a strip torn from his mattress cover. I was able to get him comfortable with the flashlight, then with the tweezers, but each time I pushed the tweezers a quarter-inch up his nostril, he flinched or pulled at my hands.

After twenty minutes, I began to lose my cool, so I took him for a drive, hoping he'd sneeze it out. He didn't, and when we returned home, he peed on the living room rug, maybe anticipating further bouts with the tweezers.

That evening I tried to make it all a game: I let him hold the light, tickled him with the tweezers. I let him put the tweezers into my nose. I asked him to help by holding my hands. Several times I got the tweezers into his nostril, only to have him jerk away just as I about to touch the object lodged inside.

I asked Les to hold the light. Soon she was muttering, then shouting, then slapping Cam's hands down. Her rage was contagious: before long I too was yelling and manhandling my son. I thought of Dr. Lauschen's words: what story were we telling ourselves now?

I stepped back. "Les, this isn't working. You're really mad. Please let me do this."

She left the bathroom. We tried again, to no avail. We returned to the living room and tried there. No dice.

I explained, "Buddy, you have to hold still so Daddy can pull that thing out of your nose. If you don't hold still, we'll have to go to the doctor again and they'll have to hold you down. Now be very quiet and you can get a Coke."

"Ho'd 'till," he agreed, "ho'd 'till." And he really tried to ho'd 'till, but each time the tweezers entered his nose, he impulsively jerked back.

A neutral observer might find the whole thing funny: the frustrated, furious parents; the kid who perversely does the wrong thing over and over; the whole ludicrous idea of stuffing a piece of plastic up one's nose. But if you're one of the performers, believe me, you don't feel like laughing. After nearly an hour of this unfunny routine, I flung the tweezers down in disgust.

This time the doctor was an ENT. No sooner did Cam plop down on his waiting room couch than he wet his pants. A Rorschach stain spread on the dark green sofa, mutely announcing to future patients: "Cameron Osteen was here." Otherwise, his behavior was exemplary.

We were called into an exam room containing a leatherette elevating chair and the usual padded table. Nothing out of the ordinary—though there was an awful lot of whispering and maneuvering going on.

Enter Dr. Dugan, a bluff, tanned man in his fifties, with a trim, salt-and-pepper mustache, booming voice, and a country-club smile exuding confidence and good cheer.

"Now, Cameron, let's look at this thing in your nose," he said. Three women stood expectantly in the doorway. That's when I realized they were going to hold him down.

The three nurses approached. One said, "Dad and Mom, if you'd help hold him."

Les and I each grabbed an arm while the nurses tried to hold Cameron's head. A look of sheer animal terror flashed across his face.

"Come on, Cam," I said, "hold still. You're my big boy. You can do it!"

"You can do it!" he shouted, as a nurse gripped his chin and another grasped the back of his head.

The doctor fumbled with the gooseneck holding the light. "This darn light won't stay put."

"You can do it!" Cam shouted.

"Not to hurt," Les told him, stroking his hand. "We're just going to look."

"Just looking, Cameron," the doctor chimed in, still bobbling the light.

"You can do it!" Cam yelled, thrashing and swiveling his head from side to side like a man dodging flying objects. Then in a panic he bent down to bite the nearest hand—mine. I snatched it away just in time.

The doctor continued to fumble with the light. "This stupid gooseneck."

"You can do it!"

All at once, the injustice of the situation jolted me like an electric shock: this was my son! How could I let him be treated like this? A wave of fatherly protectiveness surged up in me. I was just about to call a halt when the doctor said, "Stop. We can't get him to hold still. There's no point in going on."

The nurses looked relieved. "Wow, is he strong," one said as she released Cam's arm.

We'd have to sedate him to remove the object from his nose. We scheduled the procedure for 9:15 the next morning.

On the drive home I shook my head. "All this for a stupid piece of plastic!" Yet I felt perversely proud: six adults couldn't hold down my twelve-year-old son. What a man!

As the evening wore on, my pride was smothered by a swarm of what-ifs: what if we couldn't get him out of the car? What if he didn't tolerate the sedative? He wasn't supposed to eat anything that morning: what if he begged for breakfast and threw a fit?

Les's boss insisted she be on hand for a big presentation the next day. Actually, he was punishing her for having missed too many days that summer—all those school visits and doctor's appointments. I gulped when she gave me the news: I would be on my own.

On the way out the door, Les hugged Cam and said, "Daddy's going with you to the doctor. He'll put you to sleep so they can fix the nose!"

She smiled at me wanly. "Call me as soon as it's over."

The surgical waiting room at Baltimore General Hospital opens onto a wide, busy corridor leading to the cafeteria and offices. While I sat at the reception desk answering questions about Cam's medical history, he quietly kneeled on the carpet and tore a shoelace apart. Gauzy bits of string accumulated near him like nutshells around a busy squirrel. One lady asked, "What are all these little strings?" but most people studiously ignored him. A man walking down the corridor, however, caught sight of Cam as he rounded the corner and craned awkwardly to keep the boy in view. I felt like shouting, "Watch out, pal, you're going to strain your neck."

After ten minutes, the unwanted attention and implicit judgment in the crowded waiting room grew burdensome, so we went for a walk, returning just in time to be called into the pre-op area. We sat in the last of five cubicles, where a nurse asked me about Cam's medical history and handed me a hat, booties, and hospital gown—a royal blue affair decorated with miniature flowers. Cam wanted to tear the flimsy gown but kept pulling the hat down over his face. "Hoo, hoo," he said, giggling.

The minutes dragged on, but Cameron remained patient and compliant. Maybe he enjoyed all the attention. I hadn't explained anything to him yet and wasn't sure if I should, but I finally took a big breath and said, "Buddy, listen now. The doctor will put you to sleep. He'll fix your nose, and then you'll wake up. After that we'll go home. Do you understand?"

No response.

"Cam, do you understand?" He glanced at me, pulled on the gown.

"'Stand.'"

Ten more minutes elapsed, then we were approached by a tall African American man with a small mustache—the anesthesiologist. Lisping slightly, he again asked about Cam's medical history and allergies.

"Would he tolerate having a mask on his face?"

"I doubt it. He'd probably try to pull it off." I foresaw an OR wrestling match: Cam screaming, yanking out the anesthesia lines, kicking nurses.

"Will he drink some medicine if I give it to him in a cup?"

"Yes, I think so."

Two more nurses entered our cubicle in five-minute intervals, each asking the same questions about allergies and drugs. Didn't they have a chart?

All the medical personnel were coolly solicitous. If they thought we were odd, they didn't show it. But already an hour had passed and nothing had happened. Cam was calm as could be; I was almost jumping out of my shoes with anxiety.

At last the anesthesiologist brought a liquid sedative in a tiny paper cup. "Have him drink it all," he said. "It's cherry flavored."

Cam dutifully drained the cup. Right away his eyes went glassy.

A few more minutes passed. Then yet another nurse arrived, carrying a coverall, hat, and slippers for me. As I donned them over my clothes, I recalled the last time I'd worn such attire: the day Cam was born. On that auspicious day I'd been dazed with worry, then giddy with elation. What would I have felt if I'd known what was in store?

"Look what Daddy's putting on, Cam. Isn't it silly?" He was too out of it to notice. We placed him in a wheelchair and rolled him to the OR. I helped them lay my son on the table. He looked up at me trustfully: Daddy would never let anything happen to him. I prayed his faith was justified.

The anesthesiologist slipped a mask over Cam's face and told him to take deep breaths. "Dad, you can hold his hand, if you want."

I placed my son's large hand in mine and watched his eyelids flutter and close. As he lay there looking small and vulnerable, I again flashed back to the day of his birth. I remembered standing anxiously outside the incubator, touching the glass with my finger, marveling at his tiny fingers and toes, his miniature eyes and nose. Here was my newborn son! Though overwhelmed with love, I'd also been terrified by his fragility and frustrated that I couldn't hold him.

I felt the same way now.

A tall nurse tapped me on the shoulder and ushered me out of the room. With professional compassion she asked, "Are you doing all right?" I only waved my hand back and forth. I couldn't speak: an immense block had formed in my throat.

"Is this his first surgery?"

I nodded. I wanted to say, "It's not surgery—they're just taking a stupid piece of plastic out of his nose," but couldn't get a word out. I felt foolish: the "procedure" (as they called it) was almost laughably minor, the chances of anything bad happening extremely remote. So why was I choking up? Because my son was helpless and I could not protect him. Because he trusted me completely, and I'd left him in the hands of strangers. Because this experience was a foretaste of the separation to come.

As I returned to the cubicle, I was jolted by the possibility that I might never see Cam alive again. I stopped in my tracks, seized by a powerful urge to throw open the OR doors, snatch up my sleeping child, and carry him at a dead run out of the hospital.

Instead I took off my gown, hat, and slippers and made my way to a small waiting room. An elderly man with thick glasses sat across from me, underlining passages in the *Encyclopedia of Estate Planning.* I told myself not to worry and tried to read a magazine.

Only fifteen minutes later, Dr. Dugan, dressed in scrubs, pulled me aside. "It wasn't plastic," he said. "It looks like a piece of paper or something." He handed me a pill jar containing a wad of paper as large as the last joint on my thumb. A faint smear of blood stained the last quarter-inch.

"Wow," I said, "no wonder we couldn't get it out."

"We also took a big gob of wax from his right ear and two grains of what looked like sand from the left ear." Sand? Probably rice kernels from some long-ago meal. "We fixed him up. He should be awake in two or three hours." Vastly relieved, I called Les.

"I've been trying to call for the last hour!" Her voice had a shrill edge.

"I guess I turned off the phone. But there was nothing to tell; everything went off without a hitch." I longed to say, "I sure wish you were here," but held my tongue. She didn't need more guilt cast her way.

About a half-hour later (it was now 11:30), a nurse showed me into a large open area where several patients lay in various stages of sedation. Cam was still sound asleep.

"He responded to his name and turned over," she told me. "He should be waking up soon." Why, then, had the doctor told me it would be two or three hours?

Some time during the next hour, the anesthesiologist came by. He shook Cameron's shoulder three times; the boy didn't respond at all. A look of worry crossed the doctor's face, but he quickly buried it. "Oh, he's still sleeping," he said. "The first drug makes it harder to wake up from the second one. He should be coming around very soon."

One by one, other patients woke up and left the area and another groggy bunch took their places. The room resembled a fast-food restaurant. But for me, time crawled, as I grew more and more restless and worried. After an hour and a half had passed, I rose, fully prepared to grab one of the busy nurses and implore her, "What's wrong? Should he be sleeping this long? What if he doesn't wake up? Do something!" Afraid to look like a ninny, I sat down and said nothing.

Uncomfortably, I recalled Raymond Carver's powerful story "A Small, Good Thing." A small boy gets hit by a car. Doctors reassure the parents that nothing is wrong, but the boy falls into a coma and dies without waking up. These things *do* happen, I said to myself. God, what a sick joke: Boy Perishes after Paper Is Removed from Nostril.

Dread alternated with crushing boredom as I perched on the tiny wheeled stool next to Cam's bed and tried to read the *New York Review of Books.* Every few minutes I stood and gazed down at his beatific face: he could have been three years old again. I stroked his hair and whispered softly to him, "Cambo. Cambo."

Back to my stool. Worry, worry, worry; read, read, read.

I gazed around at the other post-op patients: to our left lay an elderly, red-faced man wearing a large bandage where a carcinoma had been removed from his chest; in front of us slept a female teacher who'd had an ovarian cyst removed (the nurses had talked about it within earshot); to our right was a sixty-ish woman being treated for extreme high blood pressure; behind the curtain I heard a man's croaking voice reminiscing about his wife's stay in the hospital. They were all elderly or seriously ill. What were *we* doing here?

Their voices, however, were merely background to the room's main melody: the incessant beep, beep, beep of Cam's heartbeat on the electronic monitor. As long as that refrain continued, I reminded myself, everything was still okay.

Two p.m. came and went; I was growing frantic. I began to talk to my son. "Cam, are you there? It's time to wake up. Cam, can you hear Daddy?" He stirred and tried to open his eyes. At 2:20 I could bear no more. "Cam, want a Coke?"

"Coke," he answered. For once I was happy to hear that word.

A few minutes later a nurse led us to the release room, where Cam sat upright and drank the promised icy cup of Coke while I retrieved his clothes from beneath the bed.

"Come on, son, let's put on your pants." He pulled down the thin gown and behold—out popped a massive erection! I burst into guffaws.

"Potty," said Cam.

Cam and I strode unsteadily toward the parking garage, while ahead of us walked a mother, grandmother, and two little kids. The grandma tried unsuccessfully to control the lively two-year-old girl who kept bolting away from her. The toddler got caught in the revolving door, then galloped into the narrow street between the hospital and the garage. Unable to keep up, Grandma pleaded to nobody in particular, "Stop her, will somebody please stop her?"

I darted in front of the child and held her by the arm. "Where are you going, sweetie?" She stared wide-eyed up at the looming figure.

"Thank you," the grandmother said. I looked into her eyes, and a flash of understanding passed between us: sometimes even our best efforts aren't enough. Sometimes we have to ask others to help us protect our children.

Cam was tired and dopey the rest of the day, but that evening suddenly seemed to perk up. "I sweep," he yelled between growls. "I cry!" For the first time we could recall, he was trying to recount an experience.

Leslie stroked his arm. "Yes, honey, you were in the hospital. The doctor put you to sleep. He had to fix the nose! You fell asleep and we fixed the nose." Cam looked at her trustingly and sniffed her hair. He kept repeating, "I sweep," but little by little calmed down.

At 10 p.m. I entered his room and sat beside him on the bed. "Daddy was very proud of you today, Cam. You were a big brave boy! And everything's okay now. Mommy's here, Daddy's here, and you're home." My son put his arms out and pulled me toward him. He hugged me hard to his body and wouldn't let go.

Chapter 21

Letting Go

Love seeketh not itself to please,
Nor for itself hath any care,
But for another gives its ease
And builds a Heaven in Hell's despair.
—William Blake, "The Clod and the Pebble"

One day in August I called Les at work. "Hon, I'm having second thoughts. Cam's just so cheerful today, singing and laughing. I can't believe he'd be happier somewhere else. What if we called the school and canceled the placement?"

"Wallace, what are you thinking? Just a couple of days ago you were stomping around calling this a 'living hell.' Don't get sidetracked by guilt."

"It's not guilt," I protested. "I just. . . . I don't know if I can do this."

"I know it's hard, Bunny. But we have to do what's right for Cam!"

But even Les's optimism flickered a few days later when we examined Three Sisters' school calendar. Cam would come home for long weekends every five weeks. That was good: the visits would help us stay close to him. But there were also a two-and-a-half week Christmas break, a two-week Easter break, two weeks at home in June, and the whole month of August; in all, Cam would be at home for three months of the year. With no home program, no schedule, and little help, we'd have to readjust to the same anxiety and unstinting vigilance we were experiencing now. Cam would regress, his aggression would spike, and we'd be back in the twilight zone. Couldn't these people see how absurd this schedule was?

We briefly considered backing out but soon returned to our senses, reminding ourselves that we had to do everything possible for Cam to succeed at Three Sisters: if he didn't, off to Kansas he'd go.

Conforming or Transforming

We carefully reviewed Cam's IEP with the staff, bought supplies, filled out immunization records, physical exam questionnaires, an application to participate in Special Olympics, a dental chart, a legal release and indemnification form, an agreement to reimburse them for losses incurred as a result of, say, Cam's pounding a hole in a wall or ruining a mattress. We completed permissions for testing, a release to administer medication, a flu shot form, permissions for swimming, church, and (this one prompted baffled titters) juggling.

We also had to chuckle at the clipped, no-nonsense tone of the admissions materials, which could only be called nun-like. One letter admonished parents not to pack too many clothes, specifying exactly three (not four!) blue shirts, and declaring, "We cannot and will not be responsible for unmarked clothing." The materials suggested a quasi-military atmosphere with a low tolerance for misbehavior, or even ordinary noise or rambunctiousness. They reinforced the impression we'd taken from our visits of a quiet but strictly maintained conformity. Would this regimen discourage Cam's worst behaviors? Lord knew we'd been trying unsuccessfully to wipe them out for ten years. Who would be tougher: Cam and his autism, or these redoubtable nuns and veteran teachers?

The school needed to know that he loved *Mary Poppins,* liked "Wynken, Blynken, and Nod" at bedtime, and enjoyed long baths, so we compiled a brief "Guide to Cam," detailing his habits, needs, and quirks. But maybe what he really needed was to break these habits. And maybe Three Sisters could transform him into one of the industrious young adults we'd observed there. Perhaps he'd even take a shine to the car wash or janitorial program. We had to believe that the staff would discover and develop whatever talents and aptitudes lay hidden within our son. It was either that or succumb to paralyzing grief and guilt.

August 16 was the last day of school. Terry, Cam's aide for the past two years, was leaving the school and had said goodbye to everyone. One of Cam's therapists visited us to give Cam a farewell hug. And Dana Reeves, Cam's favorite therapist, was leaving that day as well.

She tried to maintain the routine, but Cam couldn't work and seemed sad. After they returned from a ride, he refused to come into the house. I bribed him with ice cream, but then he did something very unusual: he asked for

"Bwynkennod" in the middle of the day. I wrapped him in a blanket, gave him a hug, and recited the poem, but he was still on the verge of tears. For once, the source of his mood was not a mystery: he loved these women and would miss them.

And they loved him: why else would they endure those pinches, pulled hair, slaps, and bloodied hands? They'd fallen for his little hops, his crooked smile, his initially disconcerting but ultimately endearing habit of smelling their ears and necks. They loved his genuineness and utter lack of guile. Some of the same traits that make Cam so trying—those mood swings, that volubility, that silliness, that anger—also make him loveable.

The folks at Three Sisters had sensed these qualities. If they too could learn to love my son, perhaps their love would change him.

We loved him too. That's why we had to let them try.

Will and Will Not

Though always a picky eater, Cam had devised some idiosyncratic culinary concoctions—white rice swimming in soy sauce, cereal drowned in milk *and* orange juice, cold oatmeal with raisins and milk, mini-sandwiches made of one Cheez-it and one green olive—and usually had a healthy appetite.

But in these final weeks, food became a bone of contention. One morning as we prepared for our Saturday supermarket trip, we realized Cam hadn't eaten anything yet. If he went to the store hungry, he'd likely pull boxes of snacks from the shelves or throw a tantrum. I made him an English muffin with jelly, set out string cheese and an orange—all favorites.

"Want to go to the grocery store, Cam?"

"Store, yes."

"Okay, but you have to eat first."

I showed him the spread. He only picked at it.

"Cam, if you want to go to the store, you need to eat," I repeated—several times over the next hour—but he refused to eat. Instead he growled, gnawed on his "suckie," pressed it into my hands, pounded the walls. At 1 p.m., we still hadn't embarked.

At 2:30 Leslie returned from an errand; Cam still hadn't eaten. In her absence I'd turned off the TV, denied him a requested string, refused to let him take a ride, and presented the choice again: eat and go to the store or stay here and do nothing. But he seemed content to bounce on his bed, look out the window, clap, and shout.

"He'd rather go hungry than give in," I told her. "Jesus, what a will!"

At 4 p.m. he asked for oatmeal. We made him some, but it was now too late to visit the supermarket since it would be too crowded.

An anxious Monday followed. Eventually Cam calmed down enough to work with the therapist and get ice cream, but then he started begging for a Coke, even though he'd just left a nearly full can sitting on the kitchen table. Pacing from room to room, he pleaded and stormed for fifteen minutes.

Suddenly something gave way inside me. "You want a Coke?" I asked, flinging open the kitchen door. I pulled him from the couch and pushed him into the kitchen. "Here's your Coke. Now sit down!"

He flinched and stared at me fearfully.

"Drink it, damn it!" I picked up the glass and put it to his lips.

"Drink it!" I shouted, pouring it into his mouth. He sputtered, coughed, and started to cry. I felt oddly detached, as if I were watching someone else bully my son. "Don't want it? Okay!" I shouted. "No Coke, then!" I stalked to the sink, poured the soda down the drain and slammed the glass down on the counter. Then I hustled Cam back into the living room. He hunkered on the couch as I stood over him, huffing in rage.

"I cree! Coke," he bawled, his face a portrait of confused pain.

A wave of self-loathing engulfed me. I collapsed in sobs. "I'm sorry, Cam," I choked out. I repeated the words, hugging him tightly and stroking his hair.

"You can't eat the donuts now," Les told Cam, as we shopped for groceries a few days later. "First we have to pay for them."

Cam rose from the small table where he'd been sitting but kept his grip on the bag of donuts. As we approached the checkout line, his hand snaked out and clutched Les's shirt.

"Buddy, come on. Let's check out and go eat our donuts," I said in a stage whisper. He leaned forward and chomped on my right arm.

"Yow!" I jerked my arm away and stared at the familiar red circle forming. "That's it. We're leaving now!"

Cam dropped to his knees, then lay on the floor. We could have walked away: when he realized we wouldn't coax him, he usually got up on his own. But what if he charged one of the ladies carefully trying not to stare at the twelve-year-old sprawled near the ATM? We pulled him up and walked him to the door.

I treated my arm with a bag of frozen corn as we discussed the incident at home.

Les said, "Why didn't I just give him the stupid donuts? What did it matter?"

For ten years, Cam had been eating snacks as we traversed this store's aisles, and we'd never left without paying for everything. But a few minutes before this confrontation, a store employee had spotted Cam eating a bag of potato chips and had pointedly said to Les, "You're going to pay for those, right?" The warning had made us hyper-conscientious about the donuts. Our fear of looking conspicuous had caused an incident that *really* drew attention to us. After all these years, it was still important for us to *appear* to be good parents.

We understood then that the recent battles over food sprang from similar motives. By attempting to enforce rules, we were trying to prove we hadn't given up on him. Cam, however, insisted on being heard, on showing us he had his own feelings and preferences. He was fighting for his rights.

Maybe letting go of Cam also meant giving him a chance to become himself. In helping him do that, perhaps we were showing that we finally accepted him as he was.

Let Them Eat Cake

On August 28, I went to my office and updated my colleagues on all the schools we'd visited, and described Three Sisters. The third time I recounted the story, a colleague asked how I was feeling. I told him I was having a hard time talking about it.

"I can imagine. Then let's talk about something else."

But I couldn't talk about anything else. As I sat at my desk, revealing my hopes, sorrows, and fears, I suddenly burst into tears. I buried my face in my hands as he tactfully departed.

I hadn't cried this often since age eight. Did this mean I was handling it well, or that I wasn't handling it well?

I couldn't shake the fear that Cam would feel abandoned. We couldn't write him a letter or e-mail and he couldn't really talk on the phone. How would he know we hadn't deserted him forever?

So I decided to "treasure every moment" with Cam, fully aware of how corny it sounded and that not every moment was especially treasurable. He seemed to be doing some treasuring too: one afternoon he actually lounged outside and listened to the birds chirping and trees soughing in the breeze. He'd never done that before. Was he trying to stamp into his mind the sounds and sights of home?

The next day we discovered a new bake shop, where I bought Cam four cupcakes and ordered a German chocolate cake, the sole celebratory gesture for a milestone coming on August 29: our twentieth wedding anniversary. We didn't feel like celebrating; the long-ago wedding day seemed decidedly trivial next to our son's impending departure.

While Cam devoured two pieces of cake, Les and I ruminated about guilt. If the new arrangement failed, we could say, "See, we tried, but it didn't work." But if it did work out, we'd carry different guilt: the feeling that if we'd found a good residential school years earlier instead of stubbornly plugging away at home, Cam might already be thriving.

She reminded me that none of this mattered; all that mattered, she declared again, with that determined swing of her arm, was that Cam get a chance to "make something of himself." We decided that the anniversary cake was our family re-birthday cake—an emblem not of times past but of future promise.

Labors of Love

Labor Day arrived. Several times that week I'd tried to tell Cam that he'd be moving, but each time I'd choked up. Finally I mustered up my courage and said to him, "Cam, Mommy and Daddy love you. We love you so much that we want you to do better and learn more. So you'll be starting a new school next week. It's called Three Sisters."

Then came the hard part. "This new school is a long way away, Cam. So you won't be able to come home every night. You'll be sleeping at the school instead."

"Do you understand?"

"'Stand."

"You'll be staying there. But you'll still have Bernie and your toys and music with you. And you're going to meet lots of new friends. . . ."

He looked deeply into my eyes. I couldn't tell if he understood. I wasn't sure if I did either. But at least I no longer felt we'd failed.

Les's mother told her that Cam was "imprisoned by boredom." She was right: his circle of activities had dwindled to stims and a few toys, none of which satisfied him. Though tired of his videos, he wouldn't watch new ones.

"A Spoonful of Sugar" and "Baby Beluga" would vanish from our days, along with Cam's own wordless ditties. We wouldn't hear his angry growls, his incessant clapping, his pounding on the walls, the couch springs groaning as he bounced. The ubiquitous smell of urine would fade. The kitchen floor would no longer be an obstacle course of dried oatmeal, rice kernels, and squashed raisins. We wouldn't have to sweep up pieces of string three times a day. We could rise late on weekends, dine out, go to movies, resurrect our sex life. We'd sacrificed these things for our son; in return, we'd gained identities as the parents of an autistic child. Autism had transformed us into its creatures. Now we were about to be relieved of our disorder. How surprising it was to discover that we didn't want to be cured.

In an article in *Atlantic,* Michael Sandel argues that contemporary "hyperparenting," in which parents compulsively manage every detail of their children's lives, violates what he calls the "giftedness" of life. To appreciate children as gifts means to accept them "as they come, not as objects of our design or products of our will or instruments of our ambition." He distinguishes between transforming love, which "seeks the well-being of the child," and accepting love, which "affirms the being of the child."

For years we'd sought to transform Cam, to normalize him, reshape him to fit our world. Now we had to show that other kind of love. To do that, we had to let him go.

When Cam was born on the Fourth of July, we experienced our own little revolution. Perhaps this Labor Day would begin a second revolution, one that would bring freedom for us and for our Yankee Doodle dandy.

Independence Day

Cam started his new life just as he had twelve years earlier—by kicking and screaming.

Upon arriving at Three Sisters, he refused to get out of the car and fought with teeth, feet, and hands our attempts to remove him. We hung a length of rubber surgical tubing around his neck to give him something else to bite and started unloading bags. Suddenly he whipped off the tubing, sprang out of the car, and declared, "I'm calming down."

Now he wanted to get on with it, and he calmly strode to his dorm room and claimed a bed. After we finished unpacking, the three of us walked to the lunchroom to meet Cam's new aide, Mr. Dan, a stocky man in his thirties with a crew cut and a strong Delmarva accent. We introduced him to Cam, then Les and I departed for the new parents' meeting.

The educational director, a short, chipper lady with frosted blonde hair and bright red lipstick, urged us to enjoy our newfound liberty, emphasizing that Three Sisters would do everything possible to "enhance" our kids' lives.

The remaining staff's speeches were frequently interrupted by parents' questions. One father asked, "What's OT and PT?" A mother who had entered the room weeping asked, "Let's say my son, who's eight and emotionally disturbed, runs away. How will you discipline him?"

"Why didn't they ask these questions when they visited the place?" I whispered to Les. But they didn't really want answers; they wanted reassurance—just as I did. Anyway, who was I to feel superior? Our child was one of only two students in the whole school who required a one-on-one aide during all waking hours.

It was 1:30 and Cam hadn't taken his afternoon meds. I sneaked out of the meeting and found him on the playground, swinging with Mr. Dan. After popping Cam's pill into his mouth, I chatted with the aide.

"He sure has a strong grip," Dan said.

"Did he pinch you?"

"Just grabbed my shirt."

"Yeah, he has strong hands. I think it's from all those years of yanking on strings and cords. I'm sorry."

"No problem. That's what I'm getting paid for."

"What did you do?"

"I just talked to him real soft and got him to let go." Dan seemed a solid, patient sort; Cam would put that patience to the test.

I looked around at the other kids, recognizing Eddie, the hand-shaking boy we'd met on the first visit. Another boy who looked about fourteen approached, peering at us through thick glasses.

"Dan, Dan, Dan," he said.

"How ya doin' Barry?"

"Dan, Dan, Dan. Doin' fine. Seen the planesh."

"You went to the airport."

"Went to th' aihpoht."

"Barry loves planes," Dan explained to me.

"Did you fly on an airplane, Barry?" I asked.

"I flew on a aihplane, Dan," he said and grunted out a laugh.

Would Cam speak that well after two years here? I closed my eyes and wished hard.

Then I looked for Les. The parents' meeting had adjourned, but nobody knew her whereabouts. I roamed the hallways, glanced into the infirmary, eventually ending up where I'd started. I poked my head outside. No Les. I was thrown back to fifth grade, when I'd transferred from my small country school to a larger school in town. That first day I'd felt so lost and unloved that I'd cried on the bus ride home. Is that how would Cam would feel in coming days?

Finally a staff member escorted me back to the infirmary. There was my wife. I resisted the urge to hug her in relief. Then we found Cam on the playground and let him lead us back to his room. The parents, the advertising executive and the professor, had wandered lost through the hallways, but the intellectually disabled son who'd made this journey only once before had already figured out how to get from the playground to his room. He was making himself at home.

It was time to say goodbye. Strangely, I didn't feel like crying, and when I hugged Cam he quickly pushed me away. Leslie's eyes were wet as she kissed him, but she didn't really cry either. We'd spent the summer running a marathon. Now that we'd broken the tape, we had no energy left, even for tears. But what was there to cry about? Cam was alert and calm, ready to get on with his new life.

As we walked toward the car, I couldn't resist the urge to look back. Cameron stood at his window, gazing out at us. Beside him, Dan spoke and gestured. My son lifted his right hand and waved energetically. Then he turned from the window and walked out of the light.

Half Empty

Our house seemed cavernous and tomblike; I felt equally hollow. I couldn't concentrate and spent hours compulsively cataloguing CDs and videos. Les was simply exhausted. The night we dropped Cam off, she fell asleep at 8 p.m. and did the same every night that week.

Dr. Lauschen was bemused by the contrast: Les, he said, seemed sad, whereas I was "agitated, almost manic." He again told us we were suffering from post-traumatic stress disorder.

No, I thought, we simply have a crater at the core of our lives. How would we fill it? With hobbies? Movies? Travel? These activities seemed pointless and trivial. Cam had given our lives meaning.

That first week, we had a shaky moment at the supermarket. As I pushed the cart down the cereal aisle, I scanned the boxes of oatmeal and stopped cold. "Wow. I guess there's no need to buy 'opio.'"

"No opio!" said Les with a gasp.

I nearly fled the store bawling.

We couldn't resign ourselves to the new order until the ten-day trial period passed, and the signs were not encouraging. On the first Friday, the fourth day of the trial period, the admissions director informed us that Cam had bitten two people the night before but was now doing better. On Monday, we phoned Sister Agnes Marie, Cam's dorm supervisor, for an update. He'd tried to bite her during the weekend and the next day had grabbed a classmate's hair. He was sleeping only alternate evenings. Monday was the first day he'd passed without shredding a garment. She added, "He's a handsome boy." No doubt she felt we needed to hear something positive.

On the following Friday, the school nurse told us Cam had been sick with a cough and fever of 102. "He's not himself: he's lethargic and just wants to sleep. That's not Cam!" I grimaced: already they thought they knew him. We told ourselves he was better off at school, where a nurse was on duty twenty-four hours a day. But the best nurse in the world is no substitute for your own mom. He couldn't possibly feel as safe there as he would at home.

The next day Sister Agnes put Cam on the phone. He'd never liked phones: the only person he'd ever "talked to" was my mother, and even those "conversations"—entirely one-sided, with Grammie asking questions and Cam listening for a few seconds, echoing a couple of words and then turning away—often made him testy. Maybe the phone hurt his ear. Or maybe he didn't like listening to a disembodied voice. But this time he actually tried to talk to me.

"Cam! Hi! It's Daddy. How are you?"

"Fine," he said hoarsely.

"We miss you, doodle. Were you sick?"

Sounds of breathing. "Dawwy."

"Do you feel better?"

No answer. Sister picked up the phone. "He was listening," she said.

Les took over. "Cam, it's Mommy! Hi, honey!"

"Honey," he said. Les blushed.

"Honey," she repeated, giving me a sad smile. Then she looked startled. "Oh, well, enough of that," she laughed. Cam had pushed the phone away.

We hung up feeling uplifted and utterly bereft.

That evening we reminisced about the day Cam was born. I remembered the uncanny sensation of returning home feeling irrevocably altered yet finding everything as we'd left it. We remembered passing the days like zombies, our legs and hands going about their business while our hearts and minds remained at the hospital. We felt the same way now: our son was no longer with us, but we couldn't think about anything else.

We talked into the night, reliving our rollercoaster life with autism: the growing horror as we realized something had gone terribly wrong, the brief resurgence of hope during the first years of the Lovaas program, the meltdown of 1996 and 1997, the satisfaction of finding a new school, his improvement on Risperdal, then the mounting aggression and growing despair.

Les said, "For a couple of years, I didn't feel anything for Cam. I was so freaked out and bone-tired that I either felt mad or just numb. Then I remembered those silly horse books I used to read when I was a kid. That's when it hit me: Cam was like Fury or My Friend Flicka—a skittish horse. I decided to start treating him like one. I told myself to just give him lots of hugs and kisses; you know, just act like I loved him." Her voice trembled a little. "When I started to act like I loved him, the love came back."

My path had been rockier. First I'd had to figure out that even in his disabled condition—or maybe *because* of it—Cam mirrored my fixations, flaws, and feelings. Then I had to learn a tougher lesson: that my son *wasn't* me, but a separate person with his own needs, thoughts, and desires. Only when I started to let go of him did realize that I'd *already* lost him, that I'd buried him under my rage, frustration, and unfulfilled hope. Only when I started to accept that he was leaving, ironically, did I get him back.

Word came on Tuesday, September 18: Cam was officially a student at Three Sisters School. When Les called with the news—I was at work, and she was off for Rosh Hashanah—she could barely talk between sobs. We spent the evening careening between giddiness and grief.

The next day, entering my basement office, I glimpsed the photo of Cam taken when we'd first moved into this house. Amidst his toys and books stood our one-year-old in his bright orange shorts, grinning broadly and clapping his chubby hands. I smiled then recoiled as a powerful feeling of loss washed over me. That beautiful baby had become a miserable child and an anxious, unhappy preteen. And now we'd lost them, too.

That evening Les and I clung together on the sofa, two castaways adrift on a swelling sea. "Oh, Buddy," she said. "I just want him to find a little happiness."

Half Full

The next Sunday we called Sister Agnes Marie. In her coolly sympathetic way, she informed us that Cam had gone with the group to a zoo on Saturday. "He seems to be settling in. No more problems with sleeping. He hasn't been wetting the bed, either."

"That's just great!"

She put him on the phone. With coaching, he said, "I yuh-you" and "Miss you."

I took over. "Cam, hi! It's Daddy."

"Dawwy." Pause. "Yuh-you."

"I love you too, son. Are you having fun?"

Laughter. The sound of the phone being dropped.

"It's great to hear him sound so happy," Les told Sister Agnes.

"Yes, I think he's pretty happy. I did take the pacifier away, though."

"Good. We were just so exhausted . . ."

She interrupted. "The children do lots of things here they wouldn't at home. That's why they're here."

We hung up and hugged. He was making it!

The next day Cam's case manager told us he'd won "Student of the Week." Of course, there were only six kids in his class. Still, he had his picture displayed in the hallway and got to receive the award in front of the whole student body.

I puffed up like Foghorn Leghorn. This was the Heisman Trophy, the Purple Heart, and the Oscar all rolled into one. I pictured Cam standing among the other students in the gym, performing his trademark hop and scissors kick. No wonder he'd been so giggly on the phone!

Was it possible we'd done the right thing?

In mid-October, Cam came home for the weekend. He ate as if he hadn't seen food in weeks, tested his tramp and bed, sniffed Bernie II (we'd bought a second one for home), and reacquainted himself with the bushes. He didn't seem traumatized; we even noticed some positive changes. He was clapping more softly and yelling less often, as if he realized his behavior affected others. He also made it from Thursday to Sunday without shredding a shirt. Les and I tasted the pleasures that had been smothered by anger and stress: his "hmmms" and chuckles, his little songs, the sheer sensual joy of having a kid around. Strangely, it was during this weekend that we missed him most. Seeing him again—hearing him, smelling him, feeling him—reminded us what our decision really meant.

As the weekend passed, he lapsed into old behaviors: Saturday evening brought a half-hour of raucous belching; on Sunday he stuffed a shirt label up his nostril; on Monday he peed on the carpet. We didn't care.

When we arrived at school, Cam strolled to the commons room and sank down on one of the vinyl covered settees. Dorm staffers welcomed him. "Cam-Ron! Did you have a nice weekend?" I didn't correct their mispronunciation.

Cam's teacher said, "He's doing pretty well, learning what the pictures mean, and choosing what he wants to do." I looked at the photos of Cam's classmates pinned to the wall. All girls!

"This is the first time he's had so many girls in his class," I said.

"Does he interact with them at all?" Les asked.

"Sure. He seems to like Amanda. Sometimes he holds her hand."

Tacked above the blackboard were posters with each child's name in crayon; beneath the name each student had colored a design. The girls had all chosen pastel browns and greens, but Cam had selected bold blue and red. Theirs were lightly shaded from one side to the other; his was colored over and over in an arc that turned the paper purple.

"Why is his name spelled 'Camerom?'" I asked.

"After we put up the posters, Cam went over and added the extra stroke to the 'n.' I guess he thinks his name is spelled that way," Brenda answered.

By the end of the previous summer, he'd learned to spell his name with letter cards, but hadn't moved past "Cam" to "Cameron." Apparently he knew "Cam" ends with an "m" and had fixed a "misspelling." Astonishing.

We made a note to tell them that he liked to be called "Cam." Or did he? Who was this "Camerom," anyway?

We reviewed Cam's schedule with the teacher: occupational therapy, PE, fine motor work, speech and language therapy, and, best of all, swimming twice a week. The fine motor drills might help prepare him to write, but there was no longer even a pretense of teaching him arithmetic or other academics. I knew their approach was realistic but felt a twinge of sadness.

I steeled myself for more pain as she showed us their assessments. According to them, Cam had the fine motor skills of a four-year-old and the language skills of a toddler. His functional IQ was below 40.

But what about Camerom? What was *his* IQ?

We found him in the gym, wearing a Three Sisters T-shirt that he'd already begun to shred. We gave him a farewell hug, quashing the urge to buttonhole Dan and ask why our son was sitting by himself, and left before the tears flowed.

Driving home, I broke into a chorus of "Yankee Doodle Dandy."

Epilogue

One of Us

He, who navigated with success
the dangerous river of his own birth
once more set forth

on a voyage of discovery
into the land I floated on
but could not touch to claim.
—Margaret Atwood, "Death of a Young Son by Drowning"

It's the last day of June 2008. We are celebrating Cam's birthday—his nineteenth—a few days early, because he'll be back at Three Sisters for summer school on July 4. To mark the day, I sift through photos of our son since 2001. First is a batch from 2004: a shockingly thin Cam whose medication made him vomit frequently; Cam at a hospital table, wearing a bright blue Kevlar shirt, smiling as I sing "The More We Get Together"; Cam three months later, after starting a new medication—calm, smiling, healthy. Next is a batch from 2005: a helmeted Cam riding his three-wheeler down our street; a cheerful Cam on Mother's Day; a giggly Cam in his school photo. And here is my favorite, a snapshot from his 2006 stay at summer camp—eyes closed, he swims on his back, a blissful smile lighting up his face.

Cam's life—and our life—is much better than it was in 2001. Even so, our ship has seldom found an even keel. Two different times we hunted for a new school. Once, Bright Spirit's admissions officers visited us in Baltimore. Later we flirted with a school specializing in disabled teens with behavior problems. We were put off by their use of "passive" restraints (they wrap difficult students in padded mats); they were put off by Cam's vomiting. For two years, we had to dress Cam in Kevlar to prevent him from shredding his clothes. The nadir came in 2004, when he was hospitalized for a month; yet that painful interlude yielded a medication that led to huge improvements. In 2005 he started having seizures; six months of torture ensued before we found a suitable drug.

But these peaks and valleys matter less than one fact: Three Sisters made room for our darling. They became his second family. They gave us a new life.

In this new life, Les and I are still married, partly due to Dr. Lauschen's help, but mostly due to our own determination to make it work. We fought. We cried. Most of all, we talked. And talked. Eventually we forgave ourselves and each other.

Nevertheless, we continued to ride an emotional rollercoaster. The first year after Cam left we were disoriented. Who were we? What did we like to do? After months of dining out, attending movies and social events, we discovered that we didn't miss these things nearly as much as we missed our son. During the depressed second year, I came to understand an Emily Dickinson poem that had always mystified me:

> After great pain, a formal feeling comes—
> The Nerves sit ceremonious, like Tombs—
> The Feet, mechanical, go round—. . .
> A Quartz contentment, like a stone.

In our quartz contentment we mourned both the son we'd never had—that *other* Cam, the "normal" one—and the son we had had, the one who was gone.

But he wasn't really gone: every five weeks, Cam comes home for a weekend, and he stays with us at the holidays, at spring break, and during parts of the summer. In a sense, we still live in a limbo, between past and future, between grief and relief. This feeling of dwelling *between* conditions has in fact been the hallmark of these seven years. For most of the year, we are empty nesters; but for eight to ten weeks, we're thrust back into our lives as the parents of a severely autistic child—a child who grew up while we weren't around. During one drive home, for example, I was shocked to hear Cam recite "Max wuv Ruby dah Emiwwy" in a sonorous baritone. And though in many ways he remains a preschooler, he also behaves like a typical teenager: a few months ago, for the first time in his life, he called out for "Mommy"; a couple of days later he called her a bully.

You might say we are semi-independent.

Cam may be both here *and* not here, but in the most important sense he is with us always: not only are we still consumed with his well-being, but we carry him constantly in our hearts and minds even when he's not with us physically. This has turned out to be the greatest treasure of our voyage of discovery: losing Cam has let us find him again.

He seems to know that today is his birthday: all afternoon he roams the yard anxiously, waiting for a cue, and when he sees the candle-covered cake, a look of relief crosses his face. He receives a bright blue portable DVD player, a gun that shoots bubbles, and an indoor basketball hoop to replace the old one. He's fascinated by the bubble gun and wants to shoot it himself; he also tries to operate the DVD player on his own.

Our son has definitely made progress. The bush-stripping habit has vanished. He no longer wets the bed or pees in the car. He sleeps through the night. Yet he broke two chairs today by bouncing on them and uses his new DVD player to watch the same sing-along videos he has been watching since 1991. As he watches them, he stims happily with a shoestring.

Cam is different yet the same.

Right now he's with his aide—a burly college student named Max—at Burger King, guzzling Coke and scarfing fries like any teenager. Such outings are less hazardous now: Cam is calmer and other people are more tolerant, maybe because they know more about autism. It's almost cool to be autistic these days. Since 2001, as autism diagnoses have skyrocketed, books by and about people with autism have hit the best-seller lists, and controversies about causes and cures have blanketed the media and swept the autism community. That there even *is* an autism community shows how much things have changed since Cam was a toddler. Back then, autism was considered rare, and many of the "experts" we consulted were ignorant. If he were diagnosed today, we would be afforded better services, and our ABA program would be funded by the state. But there's no guarantee—and in fact I doubt very much—that Cam would be significantly different. In any case, Les and I no longer ask "what if": to us Cam is just Cam, a person with a disability, but above all a person we love.

Maybe that's why we find ourselves unaffected by the autism wars raging today. What causes autism, whether children should be vaccinated, whether autists or "Aspies" (people with Asperger's Syndrome) should be cured or celebrated—these controversies seem to be about other children, other families. To consume ourselves with such matters would be to revert to the stage when we blamed everyone—especially ourselves—and drove ourselves to exhaustion trying to cure our son.

What matters to us now is the paucity of services for autistic adults. For if people like Cam are ever to be truly a part of our world, we must learn to accommodate them. Yet amidst all the noisy arguments about cures and causes, the best-sellers and blogs, the Camerons of the world are often forgotten. People like Cam don't create websites, maintain blogs, give interviews on talk shows, form groups, or self-advocate. Instead they get ignored. That's why I've written this book.

I've told Cam's story from my own viewpoint, yet I've also tried to speak for my son, who can't speak for himself—to convey what I believe he felt, desired, and thought. But I can't really know how it feels to be Cam. In that sense, his story may never be told.

What makes it worth telling? When we neuro-typicals see autistic people, we may think we're looking at shadow creatures, beings who share our world but aren't fully human. They live with us, but aren't like us. Yet Cam and people like him help us better understand what it means to be "normal," what it means to be a son and a father and a mother, what it means to live for another. In short, they teach us how to be human. For all of us are different from each other; we are alike in that. It is Cam's very differences, severe though they are, that make him one of us.

When I first started keeping a journal about our life with autism, I thought it would be a tale of endurance, Leslie and I as two Ishmaels who didn't defeat the white whale of autism but survived to tell the tale. By the time I finished the book, however, I understood that our story is really about acceptance: accepting Cam as he is, and learning to love him not in spite of his autism, but because of it. It also became clear that our most important lesson—and our most arduous labor of love—was to recognize that Cam is not only a part of us, but a part of the world.

When the "freaks" in Tod Browning's film chant to the trapeze artist that she's "one of us, one of us, one of us," she flinches in horror. Maybe that's how Cam felt when everyone around him chanted demands that he couldn't possibly meet. Our life with autism has often seemed an extended, amplified echo of that chant; but in our new, semi-independent life, the sound has died down enough for us to hear each other at last.

We finally accepted Cam as one of us. Then we had to stand aside and let him take his rightful place as one of you.

References

Chapter 2

Page 23: No, autism is not a death sentence, but special educator Shirley Cohen, author of *Targeting Autism,* calls it the "cancer of developmental disabilities" (10)—in other words, that it's the most serious of all—which may explain why none of the authorities we consulted would give us a diagnosis. In a brief article in the July 31, 2000, issue of *Newsweek,* Catherine Johnson, the mother of two autistic children, cites a study comparing the parents of dying children to parents of autistic children. The autistic parents were more depressed. See "The Happy Family We Set out to Be," 54.

Chapter 3

Page 24: On central coherence, see Uta Frith, *Autism: Explaining the Enigma*, 108–11, and Francesca Happé, "Why Success Is More Interesting than Failure." For examples of how even high-functioning autistic people seek local coherence, see Kamran Nazeer, *Send in the Idiots*, esp. 37–40.

Page 25: On perceptual inconstancy, see Bryna Siegel, *Helping Children with Autism Learn*, 60, and particularly Olga Bogdashina, *Sensory and Perceptual Issues in Autism and Asperger Syndrome*, 65–75.

Page 31: Some recent studies suggest that autistic children are born with smaller than average heads and brains, but experience a rapid size increase in the first year, so that by age one their brains are larger than average. At this time, normally developing brains begin pruning excess neural growth; in autistic children, the theory goes, an untrammeled growth of cells produces a tangle in the frontal lobes. Why these changes occur has yet to be determined.

Chapter 8

Page 82: Linguistic philosophers such as Charles S. Peirce would say that Cam was unable to move from the "index" (i.e., an image or illustration bearing some resemblance to the object represented) to the true symbol, which has no apparent or natural relationship to what it represents. Many autistic people are indeed more comfortable with indexic than with symbolic thinking. For a scholarly treatment of this distinction in regard to autism, see James Berger, "Alterity and Autism: Mark Haddon's *Curious Incident* in the Neurological Spectrum," 276–78.

Page 83: On central coherence, see Happé 72–73, and Frith, 109–10.

Chapter 10

Page 109: For a compelling argument that expanded diagnostic criteria explain most of the apparent autism "epidemic," see Roy R. Grinker's *Unstrange Minds,* 143–72.

The most thorough (though far from unbiased) examination of the alleged mercury/autism link is David Kirby's *Evidence of Harm.* Kirby argues that the pharmaceutical industry covered up signs that the vaccines were contaminated, and that parents of children allegedly harmed by the vaccines have ignored evidence that contradicted their beliefs. Kirby seems to believe that vaccines have contributed to the "epidemic," but even he concedes that the evidence for a direct correlation between autism and vaccines is not definitive. Since 2000, almost all reputable scientific studies have failed to prove either the thimerosal/autism link or *any* link between vaccines and autism spectrum disorders. The urge to blame autism on some single cause is not only simplistic but may also divert resources away from other research. Michael Fitzpatrick's recent *Defeating Autism: A Damaging Delusion* offers a persuasive, skeptical examination of the vaccine controversy and many biomedical interventions and explanations.

The high correlation among identical twins points to a genetic influence. If one twin is autistic, there's better than a 70 percent chance that the other will be too. And if you extend the definition to include Asperger's syndrome and milder forms of autism, the correlation is about 95 percent (see Nash, "The Secrets of Autism," 50). Yet these numbers also suggest that autism is not *entirely* determined by genes. For a medical summary of genetic research on autism, see L. Alison McInnes, "Autism Genetics Review." For a brief outline for general readers, see Margaret Pericak-Vance, "Understanding the Genetics of Autism." For an article criticizing the genetic explanation, see Chloe Silverman and Martha Herbert, "Autism and Genetics."

Chapter 11

Page 128: See Donna Williams, *Nobody Nowhere,* 61.
Page 132: James Joyce, *A Portrait of the Artist,* 7.
Page 133: For a brief treatment of executive functioning, see Siegel, 51. For more expansive discussions, see Sally Rogers and Loisa Bennetto, "Intersubjectivity in Autism," in Amy Wetherby and Barry M. Prizant's collection; and the essays in James Russell's *Autism as an Executive Disorder.*

Chapter 12

Page 137: On play, see Clara Park, *The Siege,* 265; and Siegel, 236, 238.

Chapter 13

Page 148: See Turner, "Toward an Executive Function Account," 60–61, for a chart of different types of "stims."

Page 155: For Williams's interpretation of stereotyped behaviors, see *Nobody Nowhere,* 212–16.

Page 155: On theory of mind, see Simon Baron-Cohen et al., eds., *Understanding Other Minds.* In *Autism: Explaining the Enigma,* Frith describes a famous experiment explaining this deficit (see 156–74). High-functioning autistic people often can be taught to overcome this supposed deficiency. Recently some have questioned whether the original experiments that generated this hypothesis actually measure theory of mind: see Nazeer, 71–73 for a skeptical view and 37–41 for his sympathetic perspective on local coherence.

Page 156: On executive functioning and stims, see Michelle Turner, "Toward an Executive Dysfunction Account of Repetitive Behavior in Autism," in Russell, ed., *Autism as an Executive Disorder,* 70, 80; and Christopher Jarrold, "Pretend Play in Autism: Executive Explanations," 131.

Page 156: On the "integrity" of stims, see Park, *The Siege,* 279.

Page 156: Here is the Walt Whitman poem in full:

A noiseless patient spider
I marked where on a little promontory it stood isolated,
Marked how to explore the vacant vast surrounding,
It launched forth filament, filament, filament, out of itself,
Ever unreeling them, ever tirelessly speeding them.

And you O my soul where you stand,
Surrounded, detached, in measureless oceans of space,
Ceaselessly musing, venturing, throwing, seeking the spheres to connect them,
Till the bridge you will need be formed, till the ductile anchor hold,
Till the gossamer thread you fling catch somewhere, O my soul.

Chapter 14

Page 164: See Rosemarie Garland-Thomson, "The Politics of Staring," in *Disability Studies: Enabling the Humanities,* 58–67.

Page 171: Robert Hughes, "Living with 'The Look.'" For more about Hughes and his son, see his candid, moving memoir *Running with Walker.*

Chapter 15

Page 175: Carroll, *Through the Looking-Glass,* 269.

Page 176: On echolalia, see Barry M. Prizant, Amy Wetherby, and Patrick J. Rydell, "Communication Intervention Issues," 210–11. For the chart, see Schuler and Prizant, "Echolalia," 169–73. Sacks's claims about echolalia are found in his essay, "Prodigies," in *An Anthropologist on Mars,* 233–34. Numerous examples of what Schuler and Prizant term "delayed echolalia" (164) are beautifully depicted in Paul and Judy Karasik's wonderful memoir *The Ride Together,* where they recall their brother David's meticulous recitations of entire television shows. For autistic authors' comments on echolalia, see Jasmine O'Neill, *Through the Eyes of Aliens,* 48; and Williams, *Nobody Nowhere,* 209. For a discussion of how autistic people understand language through metonymy rather than metaphor, see Kristina Chew, "Fractioned Idiom."

Page 177: Paul Collins, *Not Even Wrong,* 81.

Page 178: Sacks, *Anthropologist,* 201.

Chapter 16

Page 186: Susan Reid, "The Assessment of the Child with Autism: A Family Perspective," in Alvarez and Reid, eds., *Autism and Personality,* 18, 25, 24; Trudy Klauber, "The Significance of Trauma and Other Factors in Work with the Parents of Children with Autism," in Alvarez and Reid, eds., *Autism and Personality,* 36, 42, 43.

Page 186: Klauber, 43.

Page 190: Matthew Belmonte also advances the idea that people with autism are "human, but more so" in his essay in *Autism and Representation.*

Chapter 21

Page 252: Michael Sandel, "The Case against Perfection," 54, 56, 57.

Bibliography

Alvarez, Anne, and Susan Reid, eds. *Autism and Personality: Findings from the Tavistock Autism Workshop.* London: Routledge, 1999.

Azrin, Nathan H., and Richard M. Foxx. *Toilet Training in Less than a Day.* New York: Simon and Schuster, 1974.

Baron-Cohen, Simon, Helen Tager-Flusberg, and Donald J. Cohen, eds. *Understanding Other Minds: Perspectives from Developmental Cognitive Neuroscience.* Oxford and New York: Oxford UP, 2000.

Belmonte, Matthew K. "Human, but More So: What the Autistic Brain Tells Us about the Process of Narrative." In Osteen, ed., *Autism and Representation.* London: Routledge, 2008. 166–79.

Berger, James. "Alterity and Autism: Mark Haddon's *Curious Incident* in the Neurological Spectrum." In Osteen, ed., *Autism and Representation.* 271–88.

Bogdashina, Olga. *Sensory and Perceptual Issues in Autism and Asperger Syndrome: Different Sensory Experiences—Different Perceptual Worlds.* London: Jessica Kingsley, 2003.

Carroll, Lewis. *The Annotated Alice: Alice's Adventures in Wonderland and Through the Looking-Glass.* Ed. Martin Gardner. New York: World, 1971.

Chew, Kristina. "Fractioned Idiom: Metonymy and the Language of Autism." In Osteen, ed., *Autism and Representation.* 133–44.

Cohen, Shirley. *Targeting Autism.* Berkeley: U of California P, 1998. 2nd ed. 2003.

Collins, Paul. *Not Even Wrong: Adventures in Autism.* New York: Bloomsbury, 2004.

Fitzpatrick, Michael. *Defeating Autism: A Damaging Delusion.* London: Routledge, 2009.

Frith, Uta. *Autism: Explaining the Enigma.* London: Blackwell, 1989.

Garland-Thomson, Rosemarie. "The Politics of Staring: Visual Rhetorics of Disability in Popular Photography." In *Disability Studies: Enabling the Humanities.* Ed. Sharon L. Snyder, Brenda Jo Brueggemann, and Rosemarie Garland-Thomson. New York: MLA, 2003. 56–75.

Gernsbacher, Morton Ann. "Three Reasons Not to Believe in an Autism Epidemic." http://www.eurekalert.org/pub_releases/2005–06/bpl-trn062905.php.

Grandin, Temple, and Margaret M. Scariano. *Emergence: Labeled Autistic.* Novato, CA: Arena, 1986.

——. *Thinking in Pictures: And Other Reports from My Life with Autism.* New York: Doubleday, 1995.

Grinker, Roy Richard. *Unstrange Minds: Remapping the World of Autism.* New York: Basic Books, 2007.

Happé, Francesca. "Why Success Is More Interesting than Failure." In Richer and Coates, eds., *Autism: The Search for Coherence.* 71–74.

Hughes, Robert. "Living with 'The Look.'" *Newsweek,* September 1, 1997: 20–21.

——. *Running with Walker: A Memoir.* London: Jessica Kingsley, 2003.

Jarrold, Christopher. "Pretend Play in Autism: Executive Explanations." In Russell, ed., *Autism as an Executive Disorder.* 101–140.

Johnson, Catherine. "The Happy Family We Set out to Be." *Newsweek,* July 31, 2000: 54.

Joyce, James. *A Portrait of the Artist as a Young Man: Text, Criticism, and Notes.* Ed. Chester G. Anderson. New York: Viking, 1968.

Karasik, Paul, and Judy Karasik. *The Ride Together: A Brother and Sister's Memoir of Autism in the Family.* New York: Washington Square, 2003.

Kirby, David. *Evidence of Harm: Mercury in Vaccines and the Autism Epidemic—A Medical Controversy.* New York: St. Martin's, 2005.

Klauber, Trudy. "The Significance of Trauma and Other Factors in Work with the Parents of Children with Autism." In Alvarez and Reid, eds., *Autism and Personality.* 33–48.

Lovaas, O. Ivar. *The Autistic Child: Language Development through Behavior Modification.* New York: Irvington, 1977.

——, with Andrea Ackerman. *Teaching Developmentally Disabled Children: The Me Book.* Austin, TX: Pro-ed, 1981.

Maurice, Catherine. *Let Me Hear Your Voice: A Family's Triumph over Autism.* New York: Knopf, 1993.

McInnes, L. Alison. "Autism Genetics Review." *TEN: Trends in Evidence-Based Neuropsychiatry* 5, no. 1 (January-February 2003): 37–39.

Nash, J. Madeleine. "The Secrets of Autism." *Time,* May 6, 2002: 45–56.

Nazeer, Kamran. *Send in the Idiots: Stories from the Other Side of Autism.* New York: Bloomsbury, 2005.

Neurodiversity.com. http://www.neurodiversity.com.

O'Neill, Jasmine Lee. *Through the Eyes of Aliens: A Book about Autistic People.* London: Jessica Kingsley, 1999.

Osteen, Mark, ed. *Autism and Representation.* New York: Routledge, 2008.

Park, Clara Claiborne. *Exiting Nirvana: A Daughter's Life with Autism.* Boston: Little, Brown, 2001.

———. *The Siege: The First Eight Years of an Autistic Child.* Rev. ed. Boston: Little, Brown, 1982.

Pericak-Vance, Margaret A. "Understanding the Genetics of Autism." *Autism Advocate* 36, no. 3 (2003): 28–30.

Powers, Michael, ed. *Children with Autism: A Parents' Guide.* Rockville, MD: Woodbine House, 1989.

Prizant, Barry M., Amy M. Wetherby, and Patrick J. Rydell. "Communication Intervention Issues for Children with Autism Spectrum Disorders." In Wetherby and Prizant, eds., *Autism Spectrum Disorders.* 193–224.

Reid, Susan. "The Assessment of the Child with Autism: A Family Perspective." In Alvarez and Reid, eds., *Autism and Personality.* 13–32.

Richer, John, and Sheila Coates, eds. *Autism: The Search for Coherence.* London: Jessica Kingsley, 2001.

Rogers, Sally J., and Loisa Bennetto. "Intersubjectivity in Autism: The Roles of Imitation and Executive Function." In Wetherby and Prizant, eds., *Autism Spectrum Disorders.* 79–107.

Russell, James, ed. *Autism as an Executive Disorder.* Oxford: Oxford UP, 1997.

Sacks, Oliver. *An Anthropologist on Mars: Seven Paradoxical Tales.* New York: Knopf, 1995.

Sandel, Michael J. "The Case against Perfection." *Atlantic,* April, 2004: 51–60.

Schuler, Adriana L., and Barry M. Prizant. "Echolalia." *Communication Problems in Autism.* Ed. Eric Schopler and Gary B. Mesibov. New York: Plenum, 1985. 163–84.

Siegel, Bryna. *Helping Children with Autism Learn: Treatment Approaches for Parents and Professionals.* New York: Oxford UP, 2003.

Silverman, Chloe, and Martha Herbert. "Autism and Genetics." http://www.gene-watch.org/genewatch/articles/16–2herbert_silverman.html.

Stehli, Annabel. *The Sound of a Miracle.* New York: Avon, 1991.

Turner, Michelle. "Toward an Executive Dysfunction Account of Repetitive Behavior in Autism." In Russell, ed., *Autism as an Executive Disorder.* 57–100.

Wetherby, Amy M., and Barry M. Prizant, eds. *Autism Spectrum Disorders: A Transactional Developmental Perspective.* Baltimore: Paul H. Brookes, 2000.

Williams, Donna. *Nobody Nowhere: The Extraordinary Autobiography of an Autistic.* New York: Times Books, 1992.